IF THEY'D ONLY LISTEN

ROSEMARY SOUTHWICK
©1994, 2015

FOREWORD

What you are about to read is the story of the birth of my daughter Nancy with a life-threatening medical condition and the daily struggle of her mother to care for her. It chronicles the fight of a mother against the medical establishment; hence the title of this book: *If They'd Only Listen*. I decided to keep this account the way it was originally written, in the form of a personal journal.

Because of the sensitive nature of this material, the names of all persons, including doctors, in this book have been changed except for the following: my own, the names of my daughters Jamie and Nancy, and the names of my sisters Tina and Sharon.

It is the hope of this mother that my story will somehow be a source of hope and encouragement to others who may identify with a similar struggle in their own lives, and that they may be able to press on to fight for what they know is right, often in the face of seemingly overwhelming obstacles.

Rosemary Southwick

MARCH 1980

Thursday, March 27, 1980

We all rushed to the delivery room. I was on the stretcher. My husband Mark went to dress in a gown and the nurses quickly set me up to deliver. My doctor was paged and in a matter of minutes I was told I could push. It was 11: 37 a.m. when I heard Mark say, "There's our Nancy Patricia!" I started to cry. She was a beautiful girl with a head full of hair. It was finally over. Nancy weighed in at 7 lbs., 9 ounces and was 19 and 1/2 inches long. I was too weak to hold her, so the nurse took her to the nursery.

I was transported into the recovery room where I asked if I could lie on my stomach. It had been a long nine months since I had been able to position myself this way, and it felt good. A short time later I was brought to my room, and Mark left to go home for a rest and to call everyone in the family.

It was around 1:30 in the afternoon when I heard the babies being brought down the hall. I wasn't sure Nancy would be one of them, but I sure was ready to see her. I wasn't concerned, however, when she didn't arrive, keeping in mind that she was only two hours old.

Around 2:30 p.m. a nurse came into my room, pulled up a chair next to me, and explained that there was a problem. She told me that it wasn't until she got Nancy to the nursery that the baby turned lethargic and showed no energy. She told me that Nancy had been admitted to the Intensive Care Unit (ICU), where she was diagnosed as hypoglycemic and immediately placed on an intravenous (IV) with glucose. The nurse further told me that she had contacted Dr. Ross from the Neo-Natal Unit of Memorial Hospital, Worcester, Massachusetts. He was the consulting doctor for Hahnemann Hospital, and she informed me that he would be coming in to see Nancy. She tried to reassure me that it might only be an infection, but said that I'd have to wait and see what Dr. Ross had to say. I asked her if Nancy was diabetic. She said no, explaining that hypoglycemia was just the opposite. I was relieved, and had no other questions. She said that in case I did, to feel free to call her, or come down anytime to see her. I felt badly, but there was nothing more I could do except wait and see.

Shortly afterward, a woman came in with the forms for the birth certificate. I thought it was unusual that they asked me to sign the forms so soon, but since we had agreed on the name, I had no reservations about giving her a legal name. I could still hear her father saying, "There's our Nancy Patricia." He was so happy when she was born. . I didn't know how I was going to tell him.

Mark came in that evening around six o'clock with his parents and our three-year old daughter Jamie, all excited, of course. Jamie asked where her new sister was, and I told her she would have to wait awhile before she could go see her. She had brought the baby a little gray stuffed mouse. I told her she could show it to Nancy, and promised I would give it to Nancy to sleep with later on.

I then proceeded to tell them that there was a problem. I would have liked to talk with Mark alone, but it just couldn't be done. I was very calm when I told him what the nurse had told me. He was puzzled, since he had seen Nancy after delivery and she looked really good (although he did tell me he felt that they had taken her out of delivery rather quickly). He said he was sure that she would be all right. I held back my tears, because I didn't want everyone to worry.

My mother-in-law asked me what we were going to name her. She offered a few suggestions, and then I told her that I legally signed her name as Nancy Patricia that afternoon. You could hear a pin drop, the room got so silent. They were surprised that it had been done so quickly. Then the conversation ended.

It was now seven o'clock, and they all went down to see Nancy. I wanted to go too, but didn't. Maybe it was because I wanted Mark to see her first. I prepared them for the fact that she would have an IV in her foot so they wouldn't be startled if they saw it. ·

When they came back a short time later, they were all excited and couldn't keep from exclaiming how beautiful she was. Jamie also thought she was pretty, and you could see in her eyes how happy she was to have a baby sister. Jamie proudly told me how she had shown Nancy her mouse, and that Nancy liked it. They all left when visiting hours were over.

Friday, March 28, 1980
My father and stepmother came in during the evening hours, and I could tell that Dad was a wreck. He hates hospitals! We had a nice visit, and I updated them on what was happening. I was getting pretty good at relating what I knew to this point. After visiting hours were over, we went down to see Nancy. The parents and grandparents were the only ones allowed into the ICU, and it was only after visiting hours were over that they could see her. I knew Dad didn't like what he saw. He reassured me that she was beautiful and looked extremely well - it was just the monitors and IV that showed she had a problem. Seeing Nancy and hearing about her were two different things. She looked so good! I gave Dad a big hug and a kiss; it made everything much better. I felt closer to my dad that night and my love for him was greater than ever.

Saturday, March 29, 1980
Around 6:30 a.m., I was awakened by the pediatrician, the hospital doctor for newborns. I was still half asleep when he started talking to me about my daughter. All he had to say was that she was a very sick girl and that I should see to it that she got a very good doctor. I told him I knew, and then he simply walked out! I thought I was dreaming, but I remembered him from the birth of my daughter Jamie last time - and he hadn't impressed me then, either.

After getting my thoughts together, I realized why the hospital pediatric doctor had made that comment. Nancy's chart listed Dr. David Matthew as her "Family Practice Doctor." Dr. Matthew was a resident doctor from the Family Health Clinic, and that was probably why he didn't like the idea of treating Nancy. If he were a pediatrician, I'm sure he wouldn't have had any problem. I was not going to let it bother me; as I said, this pediatrician did not impress me anyway.

Next on the scene in came my gynecologist for the morning check and asked how I was. I asked him, "Do you know a good psychiatrist?" He pulled up a chair and sat down. I laughed, but I told him about the pediatrician and about Nancy. We talked and after awhile I felt better.

Later that morning I went down to see Nancy. As soon as I walked in and looked at her, tears came to my eyes. The nurse asked if I was okay and reported that Nancy had had a good night. But I couldn't stay. I told the nurse I simply had the "after birth blues" and that given a little time I would be all right. I cried all the way back to my room. My roommate Kate tried to cheer me up, but I told her that no matter what anyone did I would cry. I was not in control of my emotions. She said she would stick by me for the day.

Just then the phone rang. Kate answered, since I was depressed and weepy. It was for me. Although I didn't want to talk, I took the receiver. It was my mother-in-law. I explained why I was crying and said that I would be fine as soon as it wore off. I told her Nancy was still the same; there was no change. Then the bomb dropped! Apparently a nurse friend of hers had been telling her that if the doctor hadn't let me have a dry birth, Nancy would have been all right. Her friend claimed that the infection was because I had delivered dry and said that I should have had a better doctor. It was all the doctor's fault, my mother-in-law said. She couldn't have picked a worse day to tell me this. I began to yell, telling her that I had an excellent doctor and that no one was even certain it was an infection. I told her not to diagnose Nancy or to listen to people

6

who have no idea what they are talking about. I stated that Nancy was getting the best possible care anyone could give her, and commanded her not to say another word. I was worried enough just trying to comprehend everything the doctors were telling me, and told her that she was to listen only to what I had to say, and to just leave me alone! I said good-bye and hung up. Kate didn't say a word. I told her I was all right and filled her in on the other side of the conversation, which she had not been able to hear. Roommates are good to have.

Then my mother called. I told her what happened and said that although I felt badly, I certainly didn't want everyone to think I had a bad doctor. She encouraged me to call my mother-in-law and apologize, because she was just concerned and really meant well. I agreed, but I couldn't do it just yet.

After I hung up with my mother, I called my sister Tina. I wanted her to come and see me, hoping she could give my emotions a lift. She agreed to come, but would have to change her plans to spend the evening with the family at my dad's place. I then determined that I would be all right, and instead decided to settle for a good chat with her by phone. She cheered me up by telling me that my nieces had given Jamie a baby shower and that they'd had a ball. Jamie thought the "shower" meant that it must be raining outside! I laughed and my spirits were lifted. I felt better, telling her not to worry I'd be okay. I also got to talk with Jamie, and told her I would see her soon.

I then called my girlfriend Cora, who said she would be in as soon as visiting hours started. I still needed someone to come and see me. She knew she wouldn't be able to see Nancy, but being the friend she was, it didn't matter to her. After lunch, the tears were less frequent. Then a bouquet of spring flowers arrived for me; they were just beautiful. Kate was excited for me, since she knew the flowers would help me feel much better. They did, until I opened the card. It read, "To my wife and baby, I love you both, Mark." I had the biggest cry just

7

then, which Kate was sure would leave me happier. But it didn't. The first thought to enter my mind was, "How did he pay for them?" Reality set in and my tears dried up. Nothing had changed. I went down to see Nancy and told the nurses on duty that my blues were gone.

I had more company that night. I was glad to be done with the blues, because one of the visitors was a friend of mine who surely would have cried with me, and I really wouldn't have wanted that. My sister-in-law Ann came in also, and told me that her mother felt badly and had been crying most of the day. I told Ann I was sorry, and promised to call her mother in the morning and apologize. I made it clear to Ann that the apology would be for the way I had spoken to her mother. As for what I had said, it still stood that no one should say anything until I was given more information.

After our company was asked to leave by the staff, Mark and I went to visit Nancy. Just seeing her gave me all the happiness in the world. We knew deep down that everything would work out fine in time. We were counting down the ten days of antibiotics and were planning to bring Nancy home a week from Sunday. Dr. Ross came in to see Nancy and didn't really see any progress. He said that she was comfortable, and ordered that she be given the antibiotics a few more days. He saw no need to transfer her yet but promised he would be in touch. If for nothing else at this point, I could be thankful to the nurses and the doctor for their understanding and professionalism.

Mark left around 10:30 p.m., and I went back to hold and feed Nancy for a while. She refused her formula. Boy, did I pray she would take it! In that moment "alone" in the nursery I became fully aware that I would be spending every possible moment with Nancy, learning to love her more and more. It was then I decided that it was "me and you, kid" and committed myself to her.

Sunday, March 30, 1980

After breakfast, a shower, a visit with my doctor (who was very happy to see me feeling much better), and an apology by phone to my mother-in-law, I went to feed Nancy. When I got there, the nurse informed me that some lab technicians were coming up to take blood from Nancy, and therefore she could not be fed until they were done. I told her I'd wait in the hallway; it wasn't something I wanted to witness. While I was waiting, two technicians came out of the regular nursery and headed for the ICU where Nancy was. It was a young man and a girl. As they were walking past me, the girl commented to the guy, "Wait till you see this baby - she's a real sicky!" She was obviously talking about Nancy, since she was the only child in the ICU. I was furious. I would have liked to take her by the arm and ask her who she thought she was, making a statement like that! But I didn't want to create a scene, and I was afraid that if I acted the way I felt, I might say or do something I didn't mean which would make me look like a hysterical mother. So I left. I didn't want to be with Nancy when I was feeling so angry. It would not be healthy for her. I returned to my room, burning up, and told Kate what had happened. I also decided to tell one of the nurses from the nursery when they came to take Kate ' s baby. When the nurse heard my story, she assured me she would tell her supervisor and get it taken care of. She also explained that the technicians just take the blood and do not have any medical background on the patients. I told her that if it had happened yesterday morning when I was so depressed, I might not have handled it as well. I did ask that the technician be advised to keep her thoughts to herself and to refrain from discussing patients in the hallway where she could be overheard.

Later on, the nurse reported to me that her supervisor had taken care of the problem and thanked me for bringing it to their attention. I already knew the girl had been spoken to, because on my visit to see Nancy after lunch, the nurse had told me how sorry she was that I had to be subjected to a technician who had no professionalism. All I said was that I was sure she would watch herself from now on, and that at least the chance of it happening to another parent was much slimmer. Nancy still wasn't sucking on the bottle to get anything down. The only way they got any formula into her was by gavage feeding, a method which involves inserting a tube down the throat feeding directly into the stomach.

My mother came to see me in the afternoon. After a hug and a few tears, we sat and talked. My girlfriend Cora also came to see me, bringing another friend of mine. It was nice to have more company. After visiting hours were over, my mom and I went to see Nancy. My mother said she was adorable. She asked the nurse if Nancy was a little jaundiced. She was, but not enough to start her under the lights. My mother, being a nurse, told me years ago when she worked in pediatrics they never had all the equipment that they do today. She was impressed. She left shortly afterwards and let me know she would call me again tomorrow. My mother lived on Cape Cod and also worked full time, so she kept in touch mostly by phone. Everyone in the family kept close contact with me, which I appreciated. It was difficult to explain about Nancy, since no one really knew too much at this point.

Monday, March 31, 1980
Monday morning I started to put my things together to go home -- only without Nancy. I tried not to dwell on the fact that she wasn't coming home with me. Instead, I made plans to come in to see her the next day.

My doctor came in to say he would sign the release forms so I could go home. I let him know it was arranged with the nurses for my husband to pick me up when he got out of work at 4:00 p.m. That was fine with the doctor. He invited me to call him if I needed anything; otherwise he would see me in six weeks.

My family physician, Dr. Matthew, came in later that morning. He apologized for not coming in sooner, but explained that he had not been around over the weekend and therefore had not received the message until this morning. I said that we hadn't called him when I was admitted, because I was not in labor when I went in and hadn't been sure just when I would have the baby. Dr. Matthew explained to me what he could find out from Nancy's charts, promising to keep up with her progress. He also informed me that he could not treat Nancy, because he was not affiliated with the hospital, but said to call him if I had any questions about her. I thanked him, promising to let him know when she was released from the hospital.

I spent most of the afternoon with Nancy, knowing that I had to leave her and wouldn't see her until the next day. Mark came and found me all ready to leave. We went down to say good-bye to Nancy. I didn't want to leave her, but my stay was over and I had to go. Knowing that our visit with her was short, I felt tears coming down my cheeks, and I had to leave. I didn't want to be upset around her, because I felt it wasn't healthy for her. With her being so small, she needed happy people around her. The nurse reassured us that Nancy would be fine and double-checked our phone number with us. She told me I was welcome to call anytime to check on Nancy, saying, "We're here twenty-four hours!" Even if I woke up in the middle of the night, I was not to hesitate to call. I was ready to leave. I gave Nancy a kiss and left-crying, of course.

When we arrived home, my sister Tina was there waiting for us. It was nice to have her there. Jamie greeted me with a huge hug and kiss, and it felt great. It wasn't very easy to explain to Jamie why her sister wasn't home with us, but she knew Nancy was sick. That evening Mark and I made plans for the next day. Instead of dwelling on our helplessness, we made plans for what we could do to put more joy into our lives. I planned to go after lunch to see Nancy and spend the whole afternoon with her. Tina informed me that she and I were going to bingo tomorrow night and said that the girls would be staying with my dad. It was the last thing I wanted to do, but she told me I had no choice.

APRIL 1980

Tuesday, April 1, 1980
I awoke early but had rested well. I was in good spirits
because I was looking forward to seeing Nancy after lunch.
Past noontime I began to feel anxious to leave, but tried not to
let it show. Finally at 1: 45 p.m. we were all ready to go. I was
relieved to get into the car and be off.

About halfway to the hospital, I began to get really nervous.
Something did not feel right to me. Mark noticed my
uneasiness and reassured me that we were almost there,
saying that if anything was wrong with Nancy the hospital
would have called. By now I was growing certain that
something was wrong; I could feel it. I tried forcing myself to
think more positively, but the feeling would not go away. I was
glad I wasn't driving, because I would have driven well past
the speed limit to get there.

We arrived at the hospital around 2:30 p.m. The closer each
step took me to the nursery, the more relieved I felt. When we
went through the door to the nursery and turned to go to the
ICU, there were a number of people gathered at the end of the
corridor. I was concerned, but I thought they may have been
transferring another child that had been born. I tried to comfort
myself about the hospital calling if anything was wrong. There
were at least four nurses and two ambulance drivers standing
around. We passed them and turned to the doorway to the
ICU. A nurse saw us and asked if we were Nancy's parents. I
said yes, and asked what was wrong. Another nurse looked at
me and said, "We've been trying to get in touch with you." My
heart dropped. I burst into the room to see Nancy, who was in
an isolet ready to be transferred. All I could do was cry. There
were two nurses with Nancy, and they began to explain the
reason for the transfer. Apparently Nancy was still all right, but
they told me that none of the nurses could get an IV back into
her. Dr. Ross had decided that the best place for Nancy would
be in the Neo-Natal Intensive Care Unit at Memorial Hospital,
where the nurses specialized in infant care. They stressed that

this was the only reason for the transfer.

We had planned to take pictures of Nancy to show to everyone, and Mark asked if it was still possible. There wasn't any problem, since the nurses with Nancy were from Memorial and they had already started an IV on her. They gave Nancy to me to hold for a picture. I told Mark that I didn't want anyone to know I was crying. The nurses then took a picture of us both with Nancy. Then I had to go with the nurse to sign release forms. She told me they had tried calling around two o'clock (this was when I had the feeling something was wrong), but there was no answer. I explained we had left at 1: 45 p.m. to come in.

Nancy was now ready to be transferred, and I watched as she left. Inside I felt about ready to fall apart, but stayed as calm as I could. While I finished signing the papers, Mark called his workplace to let them know the reason why he would be late. We were ready to go, and we thanked the nurses and told them we would let them know how Nancy was doing when we found out anything. Again I could not stop crying; Mark didn't even try to stop me this time. All this time I never had the fear of Nancy not recovering; I just wanted to know how long this was going to take. To have a child born to you and then to watch that child struggling with pain beyond your personal control was devastating.

> 4-1-80 Hahnemann Hospital
> 20-30 minutes after birth -hypoglycemia
> Jaundice 2 days
> 4 days of antibiotics –discontinued.
> Discharged 4-1-80 to Memorial Neo-Natal. ICU

We arrived at Memorial Hospital and saw that the ambulance was already there. (Memorial was only a mile or two from Hahnemann.) We found our way to the Neo-Natal Intensive Care Unit just as the ambulance drivers were leaving. We entered the place where Nancy was, a room full of babies. Again I started crying, but I couldn't take my eyes off Nancy. I did feel better that she was there. After all, Dr. Ross did work there, and this way he would be in closer contact with her. Dr. Ross said they planned to run some more tests on Nancy since she was not responding to the antibiotics. There was a test result they were waiting for that he said would be in by Thursday. Until then, they would keep treating her the same unless there was a change. It was a "wait and see" on Nancy and he told us he would keep us fully informed.

Nancy's nurse, Mary, introduced herself and told me I could ask her any questions I might have. She gave me the phone number and told me to call anytime I wanted to. Since it was a long distance call for us, she also offered to call me when I requested it.

Mary then asked me if I would like to hold Nancy. I didn't want to. As tears flowed down my face, I told her I couldn't stay. I explained that although I had no fear for Nancy's well being, the surroundings and the change had taken its toll on me. She understood, and assured me Nancy would be well cared for.

In the meantime, a monitor had sounded an alarm and doctors and nurses were surrounding a tiny infant three beds down from Nancy. They were working very hard on this baby, and I knew it was time for us to leave. A baby was dying and we hadn't been in the room more than ten minutes. It was not a place for an upset mother to be. I gave Nancy a kiss good-bye and walked out crying. It was too much for me to take in one day. As we were leaving the hospital, I stopped at the chapel for a few minutes. I prayed for Nancy's health and my strength to carry us through this. Mark made a comment and did not come with me.

Mark and I went for a cup of coffee before he went to work. We both needed a time of quiet to talk about what had happened and what we would do. He again reassured me Nancy would be all ·right, reminding me that Thursday they would have the test results in and maybe have an answer to all this. That made me feel a lot better and we headed for his workplace.

Mark was only half an hour late (not that it was any problem - most of the day shift, including his boss, stayed until we got there). I wasn't crying! Mark walked me over to the building our friend Tom worked in, and Tom left to take me home. Of course, Tom really didn't know what to say, except, "She'll be fine, just give it some time."

When we arrived at my house, Tina came outside to meet me. I began to weep again. She asked what was wrong and I told her. She hugged me and I told her Nancy was okay, but I just couldn't stop crying. We went inside and were immediately greeted by Jamie. Although I knew Jamie didn't understand what was going on, I just hugged her and told her that mommy would be all right.

After settling down, I called the clinic to leave word for Dr. Matthew that Nancy had been transferred to Memorial. I then made myself call my mother and my mother-in-law. It was not easy to do, but they also had the right to know.

I found that plans were all set for me to go and play bingo with Tina, Diane, and two other friends. I was going to the game, but my heart was with Nancy. We left and went to my dad's place. When I saw my dad, I held back most of my tears and told him what had happened. I really didn't want to tell anyone because I had no information on what was wrong with Nancy. She had hypoglycemia and jaundice, but there was no reason why. The five of us left shortly afterwards for the bingo game.

We arrived at the hall and found some seats. Because I had forgotten to bring money along, I borrowed some from Tina. In the meantime, Diane's daughter-in-law came in. I sat there and made as much conversation as I could. However, we couldn't really talk much, because we had to keep an ear open for the numbers being called, and the place was so crowded we were sitting in the coatroom!

A little while into the game, we played a "coverall." I didn't notice I had only a few spaces to· cover on my card and I really could not have cared less. I told everyone I only had one number to go. One of my friends asked which one it was. I answered, "N-67 ." That number had already been called! I said "BINGO," and another of my friends yelled "BINGO," and I laughed for the first time since Nancy was born. A man came over and took my card to check the numbers and returned with ten ten-dollar bills. I had won $100 in cash! I sat there and was afraid to touch it for fear I was dreaming. I wasn't. I gave Tina back the money I had borrowed and said, "Now I'll have enough money for gas to travel back and forth to see Nancy." I thought perhaps my luck had changed; maybe I would get good news on Nancy tomorrow.

Well, I was the only one of us who won, but everyone was happy for me. We went back to Dad ' s for coffee and found our girls sound asleep. After going home and putting the girls to bed, I called the hospital. There was no change, but it was good to hear she was resting well. Mary also told me the nurses couldn't stay away from her because she was so cute.

Wednesday, April 2, 1980
I awoke early and made breakfast for the girls. I was feeling really good. Shortly after nine o ' clock, the phone rang. It was Dr. Matthew saying he had received my message and asking how I was. When I replied that Nancy was the same, he told me that he hadn't called to find out how Nancy was; he knew she was getting excellent care. He wanted to know how I was. I was completely taken off guard. I barely knew this doctor, having met him only twice before Nancy was born. This was amazing. He really cared about me, and I didn't' t quite know how to deal with it. I let him know I was all right and that my family was being a great help to me. Dr. Matthew then asked if I had any questions about Nancy that he could answer. I told him that they would tell me more when the test results came in the next day. Again he said I was to call anytime and to take care of myself. He promised to get back to me after he saw Nancy again. When I got off the phone, I was in partial shock.

I remarked to Tina how good it felt to have a professional person ask how you are and really mean it.

Tina and I got busy putting the house in order and getting the three girls organized because she was going to my brother's for the day. She also told me she would be leaving for home before dawn on Thursday. That was tomorrow. I didn't like that idea, but she had a husband waiting for her return and two girls whose daddy really missed them. It was time for her to think about going.

Mark and I had lunch and got ready to go to the hospital around 2 :00 p.m. Before entering the ICU, we were instructed to wash our hands well and to put a johnny over our clothing. We entered the room and saw Nancy. She was more yellowish from the jaundice than she had been yesterday, but I knew they had been putting her under the lights to treat this condition. When Mary came over, I asked her about Nancy's jaundice. She reported that the bilirubin count was down, remarking that that was a good sign.

Mary asked us if we heard about the test results, and I told her none was expected until Thursday. Well, it turned out they had come in a day early. Mary informed us that Nancy had "hypothyroidism": an under-active thyroid gland. She explained that the thyroid gland is located in the throat and is shaped like a butterfly. Nancy's was under-active. More testing was being done to see if the thyroid gland was underdeveloped -- or if there was one at all. I was scared to hear that there might not be one, but Mary assured me that a person could survive without one. They were starting Nancy on a thyroid replacement called   "synthroid." It would take a week to show a healthy response in her activity, but with the medication they had hopes that her glucose levels and lethargy would start to right themselves.

Relief came; Nancy was diagnosed. She had something explainable and treatable, and within about a week she might be able to come home! I held Nancy for a while and I felt good about her, really good.

We didn't stay much longer because I had a hard time dealing with the surroundings in the ICU. There were babies in there just fighting for breath, with tubes coming out of them. And the monitors wired to these tiny bodies made it all just too depressing for me. I noticed the empty bed three down from Nancy's; the other baby hadn't made it yesterday.

When we got home, Tina had supper all prepared for us. We told her the good news about Nancy, and of course, she was very happy. We didn't stay up late this night, because Tina was planning to leave at 5:00 in the morning for her home in New Jersey. The hospital called at 10:00 p.m. to say there was no change, but just getting the call helped me to sleep better. In the morning I heard Tina get up, so I slipped out of bed to thank her again and to see her off. I helped load the luggage and settle the two girls in the car, and off they went. This early start would get them through the heavy traffic hours to arrive home before noon. I hated to see her go. She had always meant so much to me -truly an "A-1" sister. There wasn't much more anyone could do except wait, so we promised to keep in touch.

Friday, April 4, 1980
This was Good Friday. Mark and I had decided to go to the hospital later that afternoon so I could spend more time at home with Jamie and relax a little. It felt good not having to rush. I called the hospital and found there was no change in Nancy, but it relaxed me enough to carry me through to the afternoon when I could see her.

I called Dr. Matthew to tell him about Nancy's test results. He was with a patient when I called, but would get right back to me. When he returned my call and asked how I was, I was ready this time. I replied that I was well - and saying it made me feel good, too. I told him that Nancy had been diagnosed as having an under active thyroid. I could not bring myself to

18

say hypothyroidism- not yet anyway. We talked about it, and he said he would be going in to see her and would call me after his visit. Once again he urged me to call if I had any questions.

Since Nancy had been born, everyone had proven extremely informative and helpful. The nurses and doctors couldn't do enough for our baby. They would answer any questions they could for us. They weren't just "doing their job" - they went beyond their duty. They cared and loved. I felt good about Nancy, knowing she had the best of care.

By mid-afternoon, we were getting ready to leave. Jamie was excited because she would be seeing Nancy later on when she came in with Grandma and Grandpa. After their visit with the baby, we were all planning to go out for dinner.

On the way over to the hospital, I was meditating on how much our lives were changing. There was something about Nancy that made me very proud to be her mother. I couldn't explain the reason; the feeling was just there. I did feel responsible for having brought her into the world with a problem that was yet unresolved, but I was determined to give it my best shot and to take everything one day at a time.

We arrived at the hospital around four o'clock. They had taken Nancy and put her into an isolet. (Before this she had been on a platform of some type that they also use in the unit.) She was dressed in a pink sleeper and looked beautiful.

Dr. Sims, a resident doctor we had met a few days ago, came over to talk with us. He was excited about the test results on Nancy. We asked him if this was treatable without any complications. Dr. Sims was delighted to tell us that it would be 100% treatable with thyroid replacement, and expressed that he couldn't be happier for her. The doctor said the hypoglycemia should improve once the medication started to take hold. We knew that if Nancy could eat on her own, her sugar levels would stabilize and she would be all set. Within a week they would know more. Dr. Sims was extremely happy and began to come out with all kinds of humorous expressions that made us laugh. He also said that there were other tests on her that weren't completed and said he would let us know as soon as they were received. He explained his happiness over Nancy because there are very few parents he could promise 100% recovery. In a case such as hers, his joy was overwhelming.

After talking with Dr. Sims, I pulled up the rocking chair and sat with Nancy. Even though the room was filled and the space was tight, we were still welcome to stay as long as we liked. They always liked to see the parents come in; they made us feel wanted. It wasn't very comfortable for me, though , with the monitors beeping and the staff working all around us. I would look at Nancy, then look around at the other babies, and feel guilty. Nancy looked too healthy to be in here. The other babies were tiny and sickly, with problems I couldn't begin to describe.

 I talked to the nurses about the other babies, asking how the nurses could bear the work. You did have to like the work, they told me . Even though it was hard in the beginning, they explained that it was an adjustment they made. The nurses were also mothers, and the babies were talked to, held, and loved by them. Each baby had tender, loving care; that was noticeable all around.

Before I knew it, Jamie and my in-laws were in the hall looking for us. Jamie held an Easter bunny in her arms for Nancy. I walked over to them, holding Nancy so they could see her. Although they were unable to come in, we could get close enough to communicate. Jamie didn't seem to care about what was going on around her. All she wanted was to see her baby sister. She told Nancy she had brought her a bunny and touched Nancy's hand. The beauty of being a child is so wonderful. I could see the gleam in Jamie's eyes and the pride she took in her new sister. Jamie asked about the IV in Nancy's head, and I showed it to her, explaining that she needed it so she could get better.

My mother-in-law was leaving on a trip to Europe, and this would be her last time to see Nancy before she left. I told her that the next time she would see her, Nancy should be home. It was a short visit; there was no room to move and we were all in the way. No one complained, though. I gave Nancy to her nurse and put the bunny in her crib. Jamie smiled at that.

The next three days were about the same. My visits were short, but long enough so Nancy knew I loved and cared about her. Any length of time with her would leave me feeling badly, and I didn't want to break down and cry while holding her. I was slowly beginning to accept reality.

I took Nancy's illness very calmly and didn't really ask many questions. I was comfortable with the information the doctors were giving me, and put a great deal of trust in their judgment. I really had no choice but to go along and take in what I could. I lived from day to day. After Nancy's birth, I found myself living in a world very different from what I had planned. I also had an empty feeling within me. Because of my "new world," I had to accept this, no matter what. With prayers, time, and patience, I would see this season of my life through.

Mark, on the other hand, asked questions. Sometimes I felt he asked too many; but I appreciated his forwardness, because I lacked that. I would go for days without talking to the doctors. I felt if they had anything to tell me, they would. Most of the information I needed I received from the nurses. Knowing that Nancy had a thyroid problem and was now receiving medication for it was all that mattered to me. I was there to see that she ate, and once she did that on a regular basis I knew she would be home. The more feedings I would do, the more secure I would feel about Nancy and the possibility of taking her home soon.

We spent Easter Sunday dinner at my father's, and it was nice to see everyone. I wasn't myself yet, but I did the best I could.

There wasn't much to tell anyone, but I really had no desire to say anything either. I felt guilty of something I had no real control over. Nancy was born to me for a reason, and I did not know why. Right now I was building my life around my immediate family. I would keep my home life as normal as possible and spend as much time as I could at the hospital.

Monday, April 7, 1980
Mark was working the night shift; so I would be going to the hospital around two o'clock in the afternoon to spend a few hours with Nancy, then ride home with Tom at 4:30 p.m.

We arrived at the hospital, and I sat to hold Nancy for awhile. The nurse who was taking care of Nancy had to go to the delivery room, so another nurse took over. This meant that the new nurse now had three infants to care for, and she did not look pleased.

Dr. Sims came over to talk with us, asking how Nancy was doing. I told him that if we could keep her feedings down; I would be a lot happier. He asked me if I would like to feed her. Of course, I was more than willing to do that!

It wasn't a "normal" feeding you would do for a baby. It was called "gavage feeding," in which the nurse would begin by suctioning the stomach with a tube inserted through the nasal passage or throat. (On Nancy they used the throat, but they attempted the nasal passage first, even after I told them it was too small.) By suctioning the stomach, they could tell how much food was digested from the last feeding. After the suctioning, the tube would stay in and they would attach a 1 cc syringe to the end of the tube and place the formula in the syringe. Then, by elevating the syringe enough, the formula would slowly flow down the tube and into the stomach to feed Nancy.

Even though Nancy wasn't being fed normally, I was still excited about doing it. Dr. Sims asked the nurse if she would get Nancy ready so I could feed her. She looked upset, and I had a feeling something was about to happen. The nurse took Nancy and very quickly got her ready to feed. She gave Nancy back to me, and I proceeded to feed her, holding her in one arm and the syringe in the other. Dr. Sims looked on as I began.

Before the formula even reached Nancy's stomach, she vomited all over the place. The tube came out and I got angry, to put it mildly. I knew the nurse hadn't wanted to get Nancy ready for a feeding just then and had rushed through the preparation, which resulted in a disaster for me.

Dr. Sims knew I was angry, and I questioned him on why there was also blood that came up . He answered quietly that the nurse must have hit the lining of the stomach when Nancy was suctioned. I gave Nancy back to the nurse and told Mark that he and I were leaving right then. I left for fear I would say something I would regret; that was the best way I could see to handle it. The vomiting was completely unnecessary - caused by the irritation when her stomach lining was hit during suction. It upset me all the more, knowing that every time Nancy vomited, she had to be put back on glucose water for twenty-four hours to get her to a place where she could hold down the formula. Also, she would have to be fed every hour for twenty-four hours before she could start working back up to one feeding every four hours. One feeding every four hours would mean she could go home.

Tuesday, April 8, 1980
I rode to the hospital with Mark in the morning on his way to work so I could spend the whole day with Nancy. I was determined to see that Nancy was fed properly, and the only way to do that was to go in and do it myself.

I arrived at the hospital to find that Nancy had been transferred to their Special Care Unit (SCU). I looked for her in ICU and her nurse quickly ran over to tell me she was in the next room. The nurse had been keeping an eye out for me , she said, so I wouldn't get frightened when I didn't find her.

23

Her concern was real; babies do die, and she didn't want me to worry about mine. In fact , that was the least of my worries. I knew Nancy wasn't going to die on me, even though medically she could have. I knew times were going to be hard with her for awhile, but somehow I also knew she wasn't going to die.

I went into the SCU to find Nancy sleeping. The room was much smaller, and the activity was less hectic. It was quiet, and in this nursery they would have the time to spend with Nancy for her feedings. I believe Dr. Sims knew my feelings from yesterday, and had wisely decided to transfer her. He knew I wanted to spend more time with Nancy, and I had already expressed to him what my feelings were about the ICU.

I met the nurses in the unit, and they pulled up a rocking chair for me so I could sit and hold Nancy. I felt good with her in my arms; it made me feel more a part of her. She was still on an IV, and her sugar levels were tested before every feeding. The tests were done by what they called "finger sticks." They would stick a small needle into the heel of her foot and drop a spot of blood on a strip. After a minute, the strip would give them the readings of her blood sugar level. As long as it read above 40, the nurses did not have to worry. Anything below that, however, meant they had to give her glucose intravenously.

The IV she had was a Heprin-Lock: an IV that is not running. With this arrangement, if her sugar level (glucose level) dropped below 40, they would be able to administer IV glucose immediately to bring up her level and stabilize her. Nancy's level dropped to as low as 17, which is extremely low and a severe health hazard. This level or anything below it could cause seizures.

Nancy was born with a lot of hair, and with all the IVs they had to restart her on, it was slowly disappearing. I felt badly to see most of that beautiful long hair shaved, but it was beginning to grow back in some of the areas they hadn't touched recently. The nurses told me they would do their best to keep some styling to it! In an infant, the only place they can really put an IV is in the head or the feet. Also, the veins are so tiny that it is hard to find them and to keep the IV in. Nancy had hard-to-find veins anyway.

Nancy's ten o'clock feeding was ready, and the nurse prepared her for me. She was very careful, because she had been told about the previous day's incident. In the SCU, suctioning was not necessary for every feeding , so it was just the tube feeding for her right now. I did four feedings that day (one every two hours), and she had no problem holding them down. I felt great!

They did start her on a preemie bottle, but the tube had to stay in because there was no guarantee she would eat from the bottle. I expressed my concern about the tube being down her throat while she was trying to suck on a bottle. It was difficult for her, and I felt without the tube she would eat better. Logical, yes; but the reason they couldn't do this was because if she didn't drink everything from the bottle, they would have to put it down the tube, and to insert the tube after she had eaten some from the bottle would cause her to vomit.

Wednesday through Friday of that week I was with Nancy for only a few hours each day. Mark was working nights, so I would go in around two o'clock in the afternoon and stay until Tom picked me up around 5:00 p.m.

Saturday, April 12, 1980
Again I rode in to the hospital with Mark, who was working the day shift. For the second time this week, Nancy had setbacks. She vomited again after a feeding, and I was ticked off. I spoke with Cheri, her nurse, letting her know that something had to be done. I asked her if she could make a note to all the nurses to make sure they fed Nancy slowly and burped her after every cc she took from the bottle. I had found by feeding her myself that if she was burped after every cc, she would

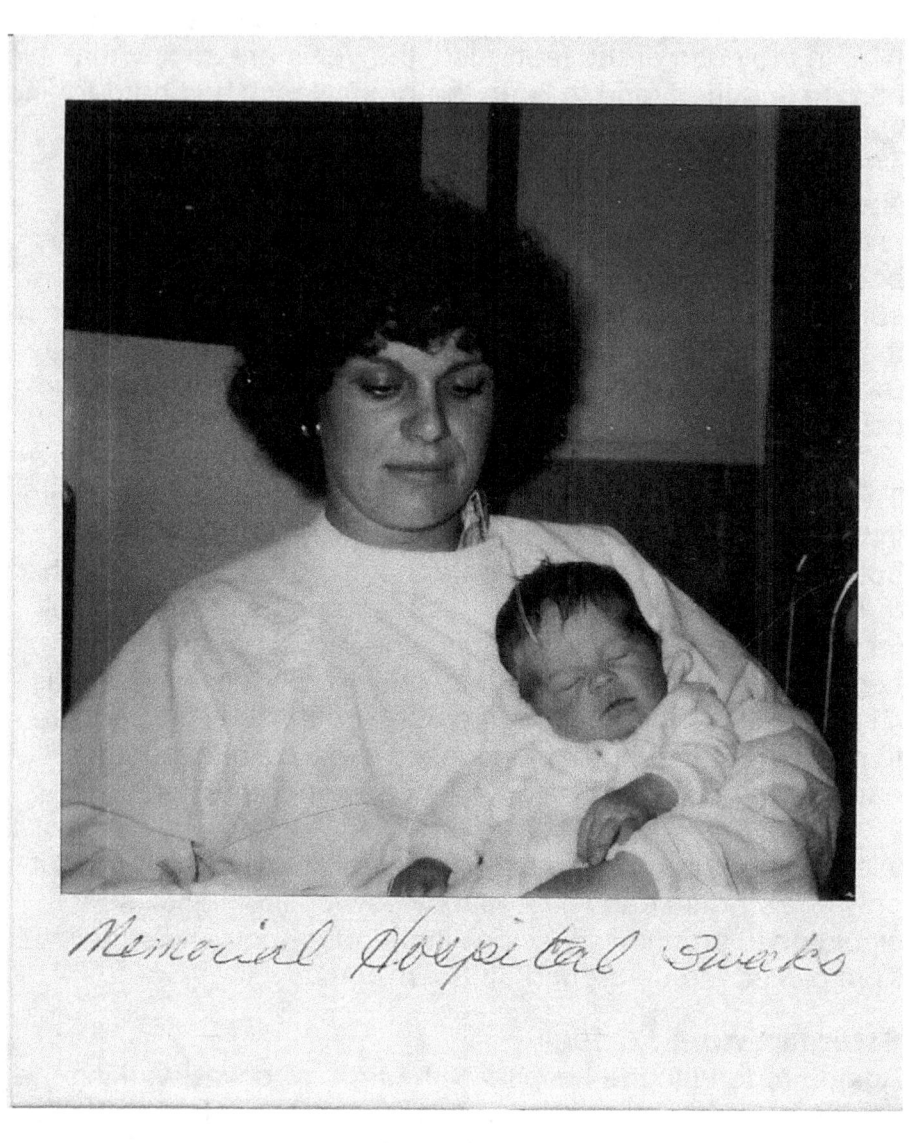

Memorial Hospital 3 weeks

MOM AND NANCY
MEMORIAL HOSPITAL: 3 weeks old

Whoever else took over would also be told, she assured me. I asked if she could put it on Nancy's chart, but was told that only doctors' orders could go into it, not mothers' notes. If there could have been a change in the policies, they would have been wise to allow mothers' orders along with doctors!

I spent Saturday and Sunday feeding Nancy, and she was doing terrific. Cheri and I were going to get her home as soon as possible. I was doing my part, and I knew that my being there for Nancy helped in every way. In the chart it would read, "Feeding done by mother," which would show the staff that the mother was coming in - proof that this mother really cared about her baby. Many of the babies did not see their mothers as much; I could observe that during the hours I spent there. The only time it got crowded in there was on Sunday afternoons. There may have been many good reasons why other mothers didn't come in very often, but I found that each time I went - no matter how long - it helped both Nancy and me. Sunday night Mark told me I was to stay home Monday all day and not go in to the hospital. I was tired and needed a break. Jamie needed me, too. I made Mark promise to go in to see Nancy after work; that way I wouldn't feel badly about staying home. Of course he was going to see her.

Monday, April 14, 1980
I called the hospital in the later part of the morning, just to reassure myself that Nancy was okay. I told them that I wouldn't be in today, but that Mark would be. I spent some time organizing things at home and enjoyed the day with Jamie. Mark was to get out of work at four, so I expected him home around 5:30 p.m. Six o'clock came and he still wasn't home, Of course, by now I was getting nervous. I was terribly anxious for him to come home and tell me he had seen Nancy and that she was just fine.

Mark finally arrived home by six-thirty and I greeted him with a quick, "Hello, how's Nancy and why are you so late?" He told me that when he went in to see Nancy, the nurse was getting

27

her ready for a feeding and let him know he was just in time to feed Nancy himself.

So he fed her and played with her for a while. I felt great knowing he had spent the time with her and got to hold her.

Mark then told me he had met a Dr. Wentworth, a specialist who wanted to speak with us about Nancy. Mark said she was a gland specialist who had been called in by Dr. Ross to check on Nancy. Mark said that he had not talked with Dr. Wentworth very long, because she wanted to meet with both of us to discuss Nancy. Mark said it had to do with the pituitary gland, but knew nothing more. We were to meet with Dr. Wentworth at five o'clock tomorrow afternoon.

Tuesday, April 15, 1980
Mark and I went in to see Nancy and to meet with Dr. Wentworth. She told us that she was an endocrinologist and that she dealt with glands in the body. She said the hospital had been in touch with her at the time Nancy had been admitted, asking her to run some tests. The reason she was called was because of the low blood sugar, which was her field. Dr. Wentworth began to explain about the testing they had run on Nancy and what they had found.

She said the main gland that controls all the other glands in the body is the pituitary gland, located in the center of the head. It is the size of a pea, and is vital to the body. The test results showed Nancy's to be under active. She would watch Nancy's growth very closely, because it would most likely be affected. Dr. Wentworth explained that the condition was treatable and advised us not to worry about it right now. She said that later, when Nancy stopped growing, she would be treated for it.

I then asked if Nancy would be a midget. Dr. Wentworth replied that four years ago they did not have the testing available for this, but today they do, and she assured me Nancy would not be a midget. She could not assure me,

28

however, that Nancy would be able to have children of her own. I told her that it was not a major concern of mine right now. When the time came, I would just have to deal with it then. I asked her what they called Nancy's diagnosis. Dr. Wentworth replied with the name hypopituitarism. What a mouthful! This would take me forever to pronounce. She also told us it was extremely rare to find this in a newborn; they aren't usually diagnosed until they are two to six years of age. More testing would be done when Nancy was older or started to show signs of no growth.

After Dr. Wentworth left, Mark and I tried to get our thoughts together and see what we had for a baby. It didn't seem as bad as it could have been, even though this growth thing was kind of strange sounding. We weren't giving up on Nancy; and we would stick by her all the way. In my heart Nancy was going to get all my attention until the time came that she didn't need me. This was not a time to throw reality out the window.

Dr. Sims came in shortly afterwards to ask us what we thought, and to see if we had any questions. I asked him more about Mrs. Wentworth (I had a hard time calling her Dr. Wentworth. All my life I had only dealt with or heard about men doctors. This was the first female one I had ever met. I automatically called her "Mrs.," but with time I would correct this.)

Dr. Sims told us that Dr. Wentworth was the only pediatric endocrinologist in Worcester and that she conducted her practice at the University of Massachusetts Medical School. He said she was a teaching professor, and very good. Mark and I agreed that we wanted to have her follow Nancy and be her doctor. Dr. Sims would let Dr. Wentworth know and set up the first appointment with her for Nancy, and would let us know when it was.

The next two weeks were about the same; life was a daily routine of home and hospital. I was going every day except Mondays. It became like second nature to me. Nancy had a few setbacks because of vomiting, and I didn't have to ask why - they knew. At least the tube did not have to be inserted, and the feedings were frequent but stable.

"How Lucky to Have Her"
Spending all this time in the hospital was a good opportunity to meet many of the staff and some mothers who made my stay less monotonous. There were a lot of premature babies who came and left. There was one mother who had a child with Sudden Infant Death Syndrome (SIDS): a healthy child otherwise, but he would stop breathing on her for no apparent reason. She soon left after being trained with monitors to attach to him at home until he had grown out of it. I felt sorry for her and was glad I didn't have to do that.

I met another mother whose daughter was nine months old with multiple problems. This mother came in every day, never missing even one day of her daughter's stay. It was her only child, a girl who had been through five operations already. This little girl was mentally retarded, and had to be fed by a tube directly into the stomach. She would stop breathing when she was frightened, or sometimes for no reason at all. Nurse's ·and staff would have to be very calm around her; it took a tremendous amount of energy just to care for her. The nurses would cringe if they found out they had to take care of her during their shift, but she was the only baby they would be assigned. She was well loved and cared for, but it seemed like a never-ending battle for her; every day was a challenge.

I went to coffee one day with her mother and asked her, "How do you do it?" She just looked at me and I said, "Never mind, I guess we all do what we have to do." I felt so badly for her, but she bravely held herself up and put the bad times behind in hopes that she would have her daughter home one day. That's all she wanted - to get her home. Her daughter did go home - for one day - but it didn't work. Later I learned the little girl had died and that it was a miracle she had lived at all.

Sunday, April 27, 1980
Nancy was doing well, and talk of her going home was more frequent. She was finally up to feedings every four hours with sugar levels at 90 and stable. Dr. Sims came in to talk to me, with news that Nancy could go home tomorrow. I was overjoyed. He told me that I would have to bring her in to St. Vincent's Hospital on Tuesday for a CAT scan, and said that she could go in as an outpatient. I then asked him if she could have it done before she came home, so I wouldn't have to worry about getting her there, or about the anesthetic they would have to give her to get her to sleep during the test. He agreed, and changed the release date to Wednesday. While Dr. Sims made out the order for the CAT scan, I reminded him that he would need my signature for the ambulance transfer. I didn't want anything to delay her discharge, and he was happy I brought this to his attention. I was learning, and my common sense of order was coming out.

I then went with Dr. Sims to their lounge to discuss Nancy, what the future plans were, and questions I may have. He asked me who I was going to use for a pediatrician for Nancy. I was a little stunned at this question, and told him that Dr. Matthew from the Family Health Clinic had been following Nancy since birth and I planned on using him. Dr. Sims responded that he knew Dave Matthew, that he was a good doctor, but that he practiced family medicine, not pediatrics. With Nancy's complications, he felt it best that she be under the care of a pediatrician.

Of course this decision was up to me. I understood what he was saying, and told him that I wanted Nancy to have the best medical care possible. I would go with what he suggested, if it was best for Nancy. He suggested two pediatricians, both of whom I had heard of at one time or another. I chose Dr. West, who was located in Auburn, not too far from Worcester. It was another thing I felt I could handle. An acquaintance of mine had Dr. West and I had also heard the nurses talk highly of him. I also knew he was taking more patients. Dr. Sims told me he would set up Nancy's first appointment with Dr. West, and would let me know when it was before I left with Nancy on Wednesday. I asked if Dr. West would be informed of Nancy's medical background before the appointment. I didn't want to have to explain the first six weeks of her life to Dr. West when I saw him. Dr. Sims promised he would see to it that all of Nancy's records were transferred to Dr. West, along with an update on her condition.

I didn't know what to do about Dr. Matthew. He had been so good to me, and I felt awkward about telling him. Nancy did need special care, and if a pediatrician was what was needed, I would have to see that she got one. I would call Dr. Matthew and let him know Nancy would be home Wednesday, but I wouldn't tell him anything else right now.

Tuesday, April 29, 1980
Nancy would be having her CAT scan done in the morning, so I stayed home to get everything in order for Wednesday, her first day home. I was going in to see her later on in the afternoon, when I would recheck arrangements with the doctor.
When I arrived at the hospital, Nancy was asleep, partially because of the medication they had given her. I saw Dr. Sims, and we briefly went over what care Nancy would need at home. Not too much had to be said. I had spent plenty of time at the hospital, and knew just about all there was to know, if not more than he did. He gave me the first appointment for Nancy with Dr. West on Tuesday, May 6, 1980 at 1:00 p.m., and for Dr. Wentworth on Tuesday, May 27, 1980 at 10:00 a.m.

Dr. Sims complimented me on how I had handled myself and the care I had shown for Nancy. They don't see this as often as they would like, he said, and he knew Nancy was going to have excellent care at home. I smiled and told him she was my daughter and I would do the best I could for her. Dr. Sims ended the conversation by telling me that when Nancy left tomorrow, they would all be happy for her, knowing her parents would give her the care she needed. He said in some cases they don't feel this way.

Wednesday, April 30, 1980
Nancy's day to come home!! It was a happy day for all of us -
especially for my dad because it was his birthday. Mark had
the day off, so we would all be going in as a family to pick up
Nancy. Jamie was full of excitement to have her sister coming
home. Jamie had waited so long for me to have Nancy, and
this additional wait had been hard on my little three-and-a-half
year old. We arrived at the hospital shortly after lunch and got
Nancy all dressed and ready to leave. I felt badly that the
regular nursing staff was not on duty, because they wouldn't
have the chance to see her off. They had all said their good-
byes to her the day before. I spoke with Dr. Sims briefly, and
the paperwork for her release was completed. Nancy was all
set to go. A nurse led us down to the front entrance. It was
then that reality hit me: Nancy was really coming home. Jamie
couldn't wait to get home to hold her.

> Memorial Hospital Discharge
> 4-1-80 to 4-30-80 "Final Diagnosis"
> 1 - Newborn female
> 2 - Hypothyroidism
> 3 - ? Hypopituitarism

A Little at a Time
The rest of the week went well; Nancy was doing just fine. She
was a good baby and a pleasure to have home. Jamie was a
little disappointed because her new sister wasn't able to play
with her, but she would talk to Nancy and show her all the toys
she had for her. I explained to Jamie that when Nancy had
grown a little older she would be able to play, and then she
would be fun. Of course, Jamie wanted to know how long that
would take. When I said, "A little longer," it seemed to satisfy
her.

MAY 1980

Monday, May 5, 1980
Dr. Wentworth called me to ask how Nancy was. She also invited me to bring Nancy to a conference at UMASS Medical Center on Tuesday, the 13th of May. She explained that a doctor from the South was holding a lecture on children like Nancy, and that he was known worldwide as being tops in his field. I told her I would be honored to come and bring my baby. The chance for Nancy to be seen by a man like this one wouldn't come often. To have her deficiency known would help more doctors to gain knowledge of this medical problem.

Tuesday, May 6, 1980
Today Nancy had her first visit with Dr. West. We had to leave home by twelve noon in order to be in Auburn for her one o'clock appointment. My mother-in-law was coming with us so she could watch Jamie while Nancy and I were with the doctor. I appreciated not only her help but her company.

We arrived at the doctor's office on schedule, and they took us in right away. The doctor's nurse first made note of Nancy's length and head circumference, then her weight. She weighed in at 7 lbs., 12 oz. I was happy to see she had gained three ounces. The nurse, on the other hand, asked me how much she had weighed at birth. When I answered, "Seven pounds nine ounces," she gave me a puzzled look. I told her Dr. West was to have received word from Memorial Hospital about Nancy's condition and her six-week hospitalization. The nurse assured me that she was certain Dr. West must know about it, and said he would be in shortly. (He'd better have, because Dr. Sims told me he specialized in thyroid cases!)

After a wait of a few minutes, Dr. West entered the examination room. He introduced himself and looked over the chart the nurse had written up. Then he asked, "How much did she weigh at birth?" Definitely the wrong question. I felt like saying, "You blew it, Doc," and walking out, but of course I didn't. I repeated myself and told him that Nancy was the

34

thyroid baby Dr. Sims was supposed to have informed him about. He quickly responded, "Oh, yes, I remember now."

Bull! Not a good enough cover-up for me. Here I was, changing doctors because it was supposed to be better for Nancy, yet he didn't even have the time to look over the records that were sent to him (if they were at all) before he saw us. Dr. West had no idea what we had been through the past six weeks of Nancy's life, and here I was supposed to allow my daughter to be treated by him? Forget it! Dr. West examined Nancy while I explained her hospital stay to him. You might say I was intimidating him - I'm sure I was - but he deserved it. I was having a little fun at it, too. I asked him about Nancy's thyroid medicine, then we talked briefly about her low blood sugar. I knew more than he did at this point, so the information we discussed was not new to me, at least.

Dr. West was a nice man and I knew he was a good doctor - but not for Nancy. He was a "pediatrician" who took care of normal children. I'm sure he did it very well, too; but for the distance and time spent on one visit I didn't want to continue with him as Nancy's doctor.

After the doctor left, the nurse came back in to give Nancy a shot and drink, her DPT and OPV .She told me to give her some Tylenol when I got home and watch for a temperature. I got Nancy dressed and went out to the office area, where I paid for the visit and received another appointment. I took the appointment, knowing very well I wasn't coming back. I didn't want to say anything about it then, however; I was too upset.

As we headed home, I explained to my mother-in-law what had happened. I let her know I had no plans to travel a total of three hours just to feel I was a number. Perhaps I had been so well informed by my previous doctors that with Dr. West I missed the T.L.C. I had come to expect. It bothered me that I didn't even get a "How are you?" Dr. Matthew, on the other hand, cared how we were - the whole family, not just Nancy. This was when I realized that a pediatrician is for children only, while a family doctor is for the whole family. That was what I needed.

We arrived home at three o'clock (I had left at twelve!). I decided to call Dr. Wentworth to ask her if it was okay not to go to Dr. West. I knew I wasn't going back, but was seeking approval from Dr. Wentworth in case there was a slight chance I was wrong. When I called, I gave Dr. Wentworth my reasons for not wanting to continue with Dr. West. She replied that he was an excellent pediatrician and said she was sure he would be a fine doctor for Nancy, urging me to reconsider my decision. I told her I would try him again and get back to her to let her know how it was going.

Still feeling frustrated and burnt, I called my mother. After I recounted what had happened and how I felt, she encouraged me to do what was best for Nancy and for myself. "You do what you feel is right, dear," Mom said. I agreed. I let her know I was going back to Dr. Matthew, and I felt good about that decision.

Wednesday, May 7, 1980
I called Dr. West's office at nine o'clock and canceled Nancy's appointment for June. I was asked if I wanted to reschedule, but I said no, Nancy would not be coming back, and thanked her anyway. I was relieved to get that done, and felt one hundred percent better. I then placed a call to the Family Health Clinic to make an appointment for Nancy with Dr. Matthew. I was to see him with Nancy on Monday, May 12, at 2:45 p.m.

My morning was turning out well. I was feeling terrific except for the prospect of calling Dr. Wentworth. She already knew how I felt, but I was nervous about calling. When I did make the call, she was nice about my decision. Although I could tell she would have liked for me to stay with Dr. West, her approval made my decision feel a lot better. So I gave her Dr. Matthew's name and phone number, and she agreed that from now on she would contact him regarding Nancy.

I was in seventh heaven the rest of the day. The only thing left was to tell Dr. Matthew what happened, and that wasn't anything that bothered me much. The weekend was coming up, and I was getting everything ready for Nancy's christening on Sunday. My sister Tina and her family were coming from New Jersey on Friday to stay with us for the weekend. I was looking forward to seeing Tina again.

Friday, May 9, 1980
Tina and Paul, along with their girls, arrived in the morning around ten o'clock. We sure were glad to see each other. They all went right in to see Nancy, which made me feel good. Although the weekend would be busy and hectic, it would be special time spent with my family.

Sunday, May 11, 1980
It was Mother's Day and Nancy's christening day- a special day for both of us. Though the events of the past seven weeks had been totally unexpected, I had really learned what it is to be a mother.

Everyone arrived around two o'clock, and we all had a nice time. Nancy was passed around and showered with a lot of love during the day. Around suppertime, Tina had to leave. I hated to see her go. Tina was not just a sister; she filled me with love and understanding, and I really needed that. As a sister and friend, she could always be counted on. It was a good feeling.

Monday, May 12, 1980
Today was the day Nancy would see Dr. Matthew for a "well baby check." Her appointment was for 2:45 p.m. I was really anxious for him to see her. It had already been two weeks since she had left the hospital, and I couldn't remember the last time he had seen her.

We arrived at the clinic and the nurse took us into the waiting area where they weighed, measured, and recorded all the information needed for the doctor. It wasn't my first time there; I recognized some of the staff people from my previous visits with Jamie. The nurses loved the little babies, and were all checking Nancy out and commenting how adorable she was.

Dr. Matthew came out to greet us and took us into his office. The nurse had weighed Nancy with her Pamper on, so he took Nancy back to the scale without a Pamper to get a more exact weight. Nancy weighed 8 lbs. 8 oz. and was 21 inches long. Since birth she had grown 1 1/2 inches, so we were pleased with her growth. Nancy's weight was also important, so he wanted to get the most exact reading possible.

After examining her and remarking how well she looked, we talked. I told him Nancy was eating very well and had gone up to eight hours at night between feedings. Dr. Matthew said that was all right, but said that he would like to do a Fasting Blood Sugar (FBS) test on her to make sure she was able to go that long without getting hypoglycemic. I told him I had been assuming that if Nancy was hungry; she would wake up and cry. If she didn't wake up, I had thought she must be fine. He then explained that with hypoglycemia, the baby would not wake up if hungry, but would go directly into a hypoglycemic seizure.

This news was enlightening, to say the least. I did know what to expect when Nancy's sugars were low, but I hadn't realized I wasn't supposed to let her go on her own. He reassured me it was all right since she had been fine up to now, but by doing the FBS test we would know more. There was a possibility it had resolved itself. We knew that her sugars would improve as she got older, but until then she would have to be checked. Dr. Matthew instructed me to make an appointment with the lab on a morning that he would be in, making sure to feed Nancy at 12:30 a.m. on the morning of the test. Then, when the lab opened at 8:30 a.m., we were to come in to begin the eight-hour FBS.

Since Nancy had been given her DPT and OPV at Dr. West's

office, Dr. Matthew asked about how she had reacted to the shot. I told him she did very well; there had been no temperature and no fussiness. He said he would prefer to give them separately to Nancy so it wouldn't be a cause of extra stress to her.

I then explained what had led me to see Dr. West in the first place. He assured me it was all right and didn't want me to feel badly about it. I told him I had the feeling I had been used, as if Dr. West needed more patients,· so I was told to get the "best" for Nancy. He informed me that Dr. Sims (who was the one who had recommended Dr. West to me) was only an intern at Memorial, adding that although Dr. West was a good pediatrician, he had only recently opened up his practice. Just what I thought: a lesson well learned.

Tuesday, May 13, 1980
Nancy and I showed up at the UMASS Medical School for the conference Dr. Wentworth had invited us to attend. Dr. Wentworth's secretary met me at the front office and led us to the conference room. We were made to wait in the hallway for a while; then Dr. Wentworth came out and brought us inside the room.

When I walked in, I saw a classroom full of medical students. I recognized a few of them from Nancy's stay in Memorial. Dr. Wentworth had me stand in front of the class while the instructing doctor examined Nancy's leg. He told the students that this mottling on her limbs was very typical of the hypothyroid child. As he removed his hand from her leg, her bootie fell off. After an attempt to replace it, he handed it to me, saying, "Mothers do it better."

That was it. I left, Dr. Wentworth said her thank-you, and I went home. If they only understood what I had gone through to get Nancy and myself ready just to get there. I had expected more information for my own knowledge, but it just didn't happen. That was okay. If another "opportunity" like that came up, I would certainly be less likely to volunteer so quickly.

Thursday, May 15, 1980
I saw my gynecologist for my six-week checkup. Everything was fine, except he felt I had lost too much weight too soon. I had lost all of the twenty-five pounds I had gained with Nancy. I filled him in about her condition and all that had gone on. After we had spoken for a while, he asked me to let him know if there was anything he could do. Otherwise, he would see me in a year.

Tuesday, May 27, 1980
Nancy had her first appointment with Dr. Wentworth this morning at 10:00 a.m. at the University Pediatric Clinic. Before we could see her, we had to arrive at the hospital early to get Nancy's outpatient paperwork done.

When I had found my way to the clinic, the nurses greeted us and led us to an examining room to get ready for the doctor. When Dr. Wentworth came in, we sat and talked first. She was happy to see how well Nancy looked. She asked how her feedings were going, and I told her she had gone up to eight hours between feedings with no signs of sweating or lethargy. I also told her that Dr. Matthew would be doing an FBS on Thursday to check her sugar levels at eight hours. Dr. 'Wentworth was pleased to hear that, and I told her she would receive the test results from him.

Dr. Wentworth advised me that Nancy may need steroids when under stress, saying that she would give me a prescription for hydrocortisone. She explained that under stress, Nancy may not produce enough steroids on her own, so we would have to supply her system with them. She explained that steroids are naturally produced by the body because they are needed during times of stress, but with Nancy there was no certainty how much her body could produce. Dr.Wentworth was sure she would need them.

I asked what kind of stress would cause her to need the

hydrocortisone. She replied that when we have a cold, we produce steroids to help us fight what is going on in our system. She went on to discuss how steroids are only produced while we are sleeping, which is why a person who is fighting a cold always feels a lot better when he wakes up in the morning. But by nighttime the system is drained of them and the patient feels worse. "So," I asked, "normally when we have stress in our body, we use up the steroids during the day and therefore need more rest?" She said yes. I asked if Nancy should be examined before giving her the hydrocortisone, and she said yes, that she would contact Dr. Matthew with instructions about the dosage and any other information he may need. I understood most of this·- especially that Nancy was only to get this medication when directed by a doctor.

Dr. Wentworth also advised me that hydrocortisone would stunt growth, which in Nancy's case we did not want to do. This is why it would have to be given carefully. She then examined Nancy, checking and rechecking her height. Nancy was growing, and Dr. Wentworth was glad to see this, but said at some point Nancy may stop and she would have to watch her closely. She commented that her skin tone was nice, and not dry. I didn't understand what was unusual about that, since all babies have soft skin. Then she explained that in children with hypothyroidism, if enough thyroid replacement is not given, they could develop very dry skin and coarse hair.

After the examination, Dr. Wentworth said they would need to take blood from Nancy before we left. This was not something I was looking forward to. I asked if they had someone really good here, and she assured me they were good. Taking blood from Nancy's veins was like getting water out of a rock, but it had to be done.

A lab technician came into the room. The nurse was going to help her by holding Nancy. The nurse asked me if I cared to leave while they did it, but I said no. The nurse looked as if she wanted me to go, but I felt that if Nancy would be going through any pain, I would stay with her and let her know I cared.

Well, the technician tried, three times. With every try, I held my breath and prayed she would hit a vein. After no success, they had to find someone else to try. By this time an hour had passed, and my strength was fading. Dr. Wentworth came in and said although she had not done this for some time, she would try herself. I felt better about this until the nurse informed me that Dr. Wentworth was going to take the blood from a vein in her neck. I thanked her for warning me and told her I would wait outside.

I stood outside the closed door and listened to Nancy scream. Tears formed in my eyes. I just wanted to pick Nancy up and leave. When the door opened, I thought it was all over; but again they had got nothing. Dr. Wentworth apologized, saying she knew of a doctor at the hospital whom she would call to see if he would come down and try. She told me if he couldn't get it, no one could. Two hours had already gone by, and I was mentally exhausted. I had already been there for a total of three hours.

While we waited for this doctor to show up, I calmed Nancy down and gave her a bottle. She had definitely used up more energy this morning, and now it was her feeding time. She had four marks on her already from the needles: one in her head, one in her neck, and one in each arm. I was wondering where this guy was going to stick her.

A half hour went by and the doctor came in. He was very pleasant and cheerful. I told him he was next, and that if he got the blood I would be forever grateful. I laid Nancy down on the table, and as soon as he started looking for a vein she cried. She knew what was going to happen. He found a vein on her head - the right side of her upper forehead. I stayed this time, and watched Nancy get her hair shaved off again in that spot. For all the hair she had lost, she still didn't look that bad. Well, one shot went in and bingo! He hit it just right. Relief was written on all our faces. He hadn't been there even ten minutes and he was already done. I asked him if he would be around the next time, and he told me to just have them call. I thanked him and we got ready to go.

Four hours had passed, and we were finally leaving. It had been a very tough day on Nancy; I was so sorry she had to be put through all of this. I prayed the next time would be better.

Thursday, May 29, 1980
I fed Nancy at 12:30 a.m. It would be her last feeding for a long while, since she was scheduled to have the fasting blood sugar test at the clinic at 8:30 a.m. We arrived on time, just as the clinic opened, and sat in the waiting room for the technician to come and get us. I was getting nervous because Nancy had now gone past eight hours without being fed, and minutes for her could mean everything. I had been watching Nancy carefully, and sighed with relief when the technician came down the hall.

But it was another woman in the waiting room she looked at. When she called on her to come in, my heart stopped. Now I had to wait even longer. The woman made a comment to the · technician, stating, "It's about time! I haven't eaten anything at all and I'm starving!" I had some bitter thoughts and felt like yelling at her, but of course I didn't. All I could keep thinking was, "Please hurry!"

Finally it was Nancy's turn. The time was now 8:50 a.m., and I knew Nancy's sugar levels were going to be low. I told the technician about it and she said she was sorry; she said that if she had known she would have taken us first. She took Nancy's blood by pricking her finger. As soon as she was done, I gave Nancy her bottle and sat there while she finished eating.

Shortly afterward, Dr. Matthew came out and told me that Nancy's sugar level was 38. He made it clear that she should not go over seven hours without a feeding. I then asked what was the lowest level Nancy could reach before she would have a seizure. He said he didn't know, but told me that he didn't want her to go lower than 50. Dr. Matthew also said he would like a visiting nurse to come to my house and do a finger stick fasting blood sugar on her. He felt it would be a lot easier on me, and I could count on it being done by eight hours, whereas with the clinic opening at 8:30 a.m. we could not rely on it being done in time.

JUNE 1980
As the month of June passed, it appeared that Nancy was doing very well. There were no doctor appointments this month, so things fell back into a more comfortable routine. I had to feed her every night at midnight, and would wake her again at seven for the seven-hour fasting. A normal baby at this age would have gone all night, but Nancy was not "normal," so I didn't expect this to happen soon. I could deal with it, but would have done anything to change it.

JULY 1980

Tuesday, July 1, 1980
Nancy had two appointments today; so of course I expected to wait around most of the day and be exhausted by the time we arrived home.

11:30 a.m., Dr. Wentworth, UMASS Medical Center
Dr. Wentworth was pleased with Nancy and actually seemed proud of her progress. In the course of our talk, we went over her treatments as far as thyroid medicine and the hypoglycemia. She told me she could tell just by looking at Nancy that her thyroid level was quite good. We also talked about having testing done on her in the future, at the point when Nancy might show signs that she was no longer growing on her own. For now, Dr. Wentworth would just keep a close watch on her.

I listened to what Dr. Wentworth was telling me about Nancy's growth deficiency, but I had to put it behind me for now. I was mainly concerned with her hypoglycemia at the moment, because it had to be treated daily. I couldn't let myself be concerned about something that was not immediate. I gladly took the information, but knew I would have to let it lie until Dr. Wentworth told me, "now." I was not afraid. When the time came, I would deal with it. Dr. Wentworth also told me that she would give me a letter to carry with me, describing Nancy's medical conditions and what her treatment was to be in an emergency. At any time, no matter where I might be, I could give the letter to the doctor treating her and it would ensure that Nancy got the most appropriate care.

When we were done with the visit, I went out into the waiting area and fed Nancy. By the time Nancy was done, we were ready to move on to the next appointment.

1:30 p.m., Child Development Service

Child Development Service is a program in which children born prematurely or with birth defects are screened for developmental problems. They study the child as he or she grows, picking up delays in the child's development and providing help for the child in certain areas if needed.

Nancy and I were led into a room, where again she had to be weighed and measured by the nurse. Shortly afterward a doctor came in and examined Nancy. When he was finished and had left the room, I got Nancy dressed.

Some time lapsed, then two doctors came in: the one who had examined Nancy and a second one. The new one, Dr. Samuels, introduced himself as the doctor who was actually seeing Nancy, since the other one was a resident. Then the resident proceeded to tell Dr. Samuels what he had found in examining Nancy. This was definitely a different experience for me. I was amused by it all, to say the least.

After the resident finished, Dr. Samuels wanted to examine Nancy himself, so I undressed her again. In the meantime, a girl entered the room who was going to test Nancy in the areas of a typical three-month-old child. After Dr. Samuels had examined Nancy, he asked me to put her down on a mat that was spread on the floor. As Nancy lay on the mat, the girl started some simple tests to see what Nancy could do. She had Nancy follow objects, and checked to see if she could roll over and hold her head up. Nancy passed with flying colors, and I was told she was doing well.

I was actually humored by all this, because I knew she was doing all these things. I did understand, however, that although it may sound and look ridiculous, there was good reason for this testing. They could actually tell a lot by the child's movements that we parents take for granted. We left at 4:44 p.m., and I was exhausted. I never dreamed it would take so long.

Wednesday, July 9, 1980
I had been in touch with the Town Visiting Nurses and had set up an appointment for them to come in this morning at eight o'clock to do a finger stick fasting blood sugar test on Nancy. The nurse arrived at the house just before eight, which impressed me very much. I was getting used to waiting for people, and she proved to me that some are very prompt. I brought the nurse to Nancy's room, where she was still sleeping. She hated to wake Nancy, not to mention sticking her finger with a needle. Anyway, she proceeded to test her, but it did not work. She repeated it, but failed again.

The sticks she was using had been given to me by the clinic for the visiting nurse 's convenience, but for some unknown reason they would not take. The nurse was doing it properly, because I had seen it done several times. The problem lay in the sticks, which did not register. The nurse was all apologetic, but I told her it was all right; it wasn't her fault.

It was necessary to get the test done, but I wasn't very concerned. I had been shown how to test Nancy myself, but I didn't have enough guts to do it. I felt that I did not want the nurse to get a reading on Nancy anyway, since having it fail would show that it couldn't be done in the home. I was doing all that I could for Nancy, and felt it was not my responsibility to go any further with my medical treatment of her. I was doing enough; I did not want this done in my home. I had told Dr. Matthew that I would agree to try to do the blood test myself if Nancy had a seizure at home -- but only that I would try. I never committed myself to following through.

I called Dr. Matthew later in the morning to let him know the blood test did not work and why. He instructed me to feed her at two o'clock Thursday morning and said he would have the lab do some testing on her at ten o'clock when she was brought in for her checkup. This made me feel better, and I didn't mind feeding her at 2:00 a.m.

Thursday, July 10, 1980
I fed Nancy at 2 a.m. and she was doing all right by morning and didn't seem hungry. We went along to the clinic for the ten o'clock appointment. Nancy weighed in at 10 lbs., 13 oz., and her height was 221/2 inches. When we saw Dr. Matthew, he had us go up to the lab first for the fasting blood sugar test. The lab took the blood from her finger and she didn't cry very hard. I knew this sign; her sugar levels were not going to turn up very high.

We went into Dr. Matthew's office while waiting for the results. As we talked, he mentioned that Nancy would get her DPT shot today. Then in two weeks I was to bring her back to have the OPV. Before we left, the test results came back and the reading was 42 - a good level. Dr. Matthew said she would be all right up to eight hours, and told me to watch her to see how she did.

He wanted to see her next month, but I told him we would be going on vacation the last week in July, so I would have to make her appointment for after we got back. But it turned out that he would be on vacation the first week in August, so we agreed to set her checkup for before I went away. Her last well checkup had been in May, so he didn't want her to go much longer.

Friday, July 25, 1980
Nancy had a well child checkup with Dr. Matthew. She weighed in at 12 lbs., and Dr. Matthew measured her at 24 inches long. It showed quite a difference in height within two weeks, but she had been measured by a nurse the last time, so that explained the difference. The nurses did a fine job measuring Nancy, but in order to get a more accurate measurement, the doctor would lay her down on a sheet of paper, marking it at the top of her head and at the bottom of her feet. Then he would measure between the marks on the paper. Both of Nancy's doctors were very precise regarding her height, because they were checking for any slowing of growth. Up till now she had been growing normally. The standard growth chart was also reading "normal," so it didn't take too much to get me up on cloud nine.

I received Nancy's medical letter in the mail from Dr. Wentworth. It stated:

"To whomever this may concern:

This letter will introduce you to Nancy, who is under my care for hypopituitarism. She has TSH deficiency, for which she receives thyroxine replacement, and also ACTH and growth hormone deficiency biochemically for which she is not at present receiving any treatment. Should Nancy be ill, particularly if she has a high fever, is vomiting, or dehydrated, she should receive steroid coverage in a dose of 25 - 50 mg/M2/day. This should be done sparingly and only as absolutely necessary as it may significantly impair her growth.

Please contact me if I can be of any further service.

Dr. Wentworth"

Saturday, July 26, 1980
Mark, the girls, and I left on vacation for a week's stay at Cape Cod, in the town of Eastham. We had been vacationing at the Cape for ten years now, and it had gotten boring for me. It was

always a week of total relaxation - the beach and no phone! We would leave everything behind and drink in the slow life of the Cape. This year was special to me - I really felt good and couldn't wait to get away from the everyday routine.

AUGUST 1980

Tuesday, August 12, 1980
Nancy was scheduled to see Dr. Wentworth at the Medical Center at ten o'clock. Dr. Wentworth was the one I really wanted to please with Nancy's progress. To receive her approval and encouragement was important to me. Dr. Wentworth was a brilliant doctor, and I felt that to receive her approval of my handling of Nancy was to receive an "A+" as a mother. I always felt somewhat insecure around Dr. Wentworth, because Nancy lived with me twenty-four hours a day, and I based her treatment on our home life. But as soon as I would sit down with Dr. Wentworth for Nancy's appointments, I felt like a student, not a mother. And, in fact, I was a student; I had to learn Nancy not only as a mother but as a doctor. It was getting scary; more and more responsibility was coming down on me, and I lived in fear of doing something wrong.

Dr. Wentworth came in and examined Nancy, saying that she looked really good. Then she brought a resident doctor in to meet Nancy. Approval! She carefully measured Nancy and was pleased with her growth. We also talked for awhile, and I took in what I could, asking questions when I was unsure. If there was something I really couldn't understand, I made a mental note to ask Dr. Matthew the next time I spoke to him.

I told Dr. Wentworth that Nancy was now going anywhere from ten to twelve hours overnight between feedings. Nancy was also on cereal and fruit, which was why I felt she could go longer without eating. Dr. Wentworth agreed, and was pleased that Nancy was showing progress with her blood sugar levels. Dr. Wentworth told me to give her more solid food than liquid, since the solid foods break down more slowly.

Dr. Wentworth also needed blood drawn from Nancy again, which neither the doctor nor I were too thrilled about. The memory was still there from last time. The blood was successfully drawn on the third try. The resident who did it told me he would only try three times; after that he would count himself out.

Wednesday, August 20, 1980

I got up at 7:30 a.m. to check on Nancy - she was still sleeping. I went into the kitchen to get her bottle ready and to start breakfast. She was due to eat by eight o'clock. By the time her breakfast was ready, I was growing nervous because she hadn't woken up yet.

I went into Nancy's room, picked her up, and tried to wake her, but there was no response. I quickly made my way to the kitchen, grabbed her bottle, and started to feed her. She was stretched out and lethargic, with her eyes blinking. I was truly scared. It had been drilled into my head that Nancy had to eat, and Dr. Wentworth had suggested that when Nancy showed these signs I should rub sugar around the inside of her mouth in order to get the sugar into her system as quickly as possible. I did this between her drinks from the bottle. It only took her a few minutes to stop moving her legs and arms, but it was a good ten minutes before she responded to me. I talked to her to reassure her she would be all right. The movements of her limbs were a sort of mild twitching, not erratic and not constant. When she finally became alert she seemed fine - tired, but at least she finished her breakfast. I was mentally exhausted.

At nine o'clock I called the clinic and talked with Dr. Matthew. I was very emotional over the phone, trying to hold back my tears. He told me to come in with Nancy so he could check her over.

We arrived at the clinic just before ten o'clock and Dr. Matthew was waiting for us. I gave a sigh of relief as soon as I saw him.

Just being there, I could feel the burden lift from my shoulders.

I took Nancy into the office and did the best job I could explaining exactly what had happened. Dr. Matthew checked Nancy's reflexes, vision, and alertness. Everything seemed fine. He also asked me if she seemed okay to me. I told him she seemed fine, aside from being tired. He said it sounded as though she'd had a hypoglycemic seizure. However, because he had not seen it himself and no test had been taken, he couldn't say for sure. He immediately reassured me that I had done the right thing and that she looked fine. Nancy had gone twelve hours without a feeding, so he wanted a ten-hour fast done on her in the morning and gave me the equipment to take her blood for the test.

The lab technician went over the procedure for drawing blood from Nancy. I had seen it done many times, and was very willing to do it. The procedure was to first wipe the finger with alcohol, wipe again with a sterile cotton cloth, prick it with a sterile pin, wipe it again, and squeeze the blood out - enough to fill four tiny tubes. If Nancy were to have another seizure, I was to use a dextro strip for a quick test. I said I would try to use the dextro strip, but I didn't promise. I did not have the control that would be needed to take a sugar test while Nancy was having a seizure - at least not yet. I did say that if it happened again, I would attempt it.

That evening I fed Nancy at ten o'clock so I could test her in the morning at eight for the ten-hour BFS.

Thursday, August 21, 1980
I awoke at seven-thirty and checked Nancy. She started to awaken, so I knew she was all right. I went to the kitchen and got her breakfast started, and prepared the items for taking her blood. At eight o'clock I took the blood from Nancy's finger. She cried, but it was over in no time. Right after that, I fed her and she ate really well. It was then I knew the reading of the BFS would likely be low, because she was so hungry.

Later in the morning I brought to the clinic the Microhematocrit tubes that I had filled with blood. I just dropped them off at the lab; Dr. Matthew was to call me with the results later on today.

Around mid-afternoon Dr. Matthew called. The reading was 44, and he felt that ten hours was too long for her to go without food. Forty-four was all right, but when blood sugar gets that low it can fall rapidly within a short period, so it was best to feed her within eight hours until a higher reading was found. We would wait, hoping that when she got older she would be able to go longer.

Dr. Matthew also told me he had spoken of Nancy to a Dr. Adams, a neurologist from the UMASS Medical Center. Dr. Adams agreed that it sounded as though Nancy had suffered a hypoglycemic seizure, and recommended that an E.E.G. test (brain wave test for seizure disorders) be done to see if it would tell them anything more. Dr. Matthew assured me that it would be a fairly simple test and wouldn't hurt her. They would simply attach wires to her head while she was asleep. The wires would then transmit readings of what was going on in her brain.
From what I could understand, it sounded all right to me. Dr. Matthew said he would put me through to a nurse from the clinic to set up the appointment. Before doing that, he asked if I was all right and if I had any more questions. I told him I was fine, and that I had no more questions.

Nancy had an appointment for September 10th at 8:30 a.m. at the UMASS Medical Center. I had no fear about her having the EEG testing done, but I did hope that nothing else would show up. I had enough to learn; I had no desire to learn anything else. My attitude was to go ahead and have the testing done so Nancy could prove to us that there was nothing wrong with her brain.

SEPTEMBER 1980

Wednesday, September 3, 1980
When I took my older daughter Jamie for her yearly checkup with Dr. Matthew, she passed her physical with flying colors. Dr. Matthew thought she was a pretty neat girl. She beamed from ear to ear, taking it all in. Of course she told him it was her birthday yesterday and that she was four years old.

Dr. Matthew was concerned about Jamie because of all the attention Nancy had been receiving (we had already discussed this at an earlier date). I had told him I was aware of this and that I would do my best to help Jamie understand. I would make special time just for her.

Sunday, September 7, 1980
A big day for Nancy and Mark-Nancy said "DA DA" for the first time! After all the hours a mother spends repeating "MA MA" to the baby, it never fails: "DA DA" wins. We were all thrilled, especially Jamie. She thought it was great, and took it as a big joke on me that I had wanted her to say "Mama" first.

Wednesday, September 10, 1980
Today Nancy was due at the Medical Center at 8:30 a.m. for the EEG testing. It was a very early morning for us, because we had to allow a little over half an hour for travel time. I had put Nancy to bed later than usual the previous night, waking her at six this morning so she would be tired enough to take a nap for the test. They needed her to have a natural sleep if at all possible.

The technician came out to the waiting area and escorted us to the testing room. There was a bed in the room, and off to the side in another small room sat the EEG machine that would take the reading. He darkened the room and asked me to give Nancy a bottle and see if she would go to sleep. If not, he would give her some medication. I told him Nancy would have no problem sleeping because she had almost fallen asleep in the car on the way there. Nancy quickly went to sleep, and I laid her down on the bed so the doctor could wire her up.

Carefully and without much motion, he placed some tiny cups with wires on specific areas of her head. It was interesting to watch. He had to do this quickly and quietly in order not to wake her, and to be sure there would be enough time for the test before she awoke.

The reason I never really minded taking Nancy to all these appointments was that I was learning. It was something I had never asked for, but now the choice was not mine to make. If I were to fight our circumstances, I would get nowhere and Nancy would not get the proper care. I would do what was asked and try to learn at the same time. I was becoming a nurse - a profession I would never have chosen. While pregnant with Nancy, I had often wondered what I would do with my life. I remember saying, "Big deal. I have another baby to feed and take care of, but what am I going to do? Where is my future?" I was bored, and although caring for two small children was all right, I needed something more.

Well, now that my nine-and-a-half months were over, I was definitely not going to be bored. My future was going to be very busy. I was being introduced to a field I had once feared, and to have a child whose condition represented one in a million was even more challenging. It didn't seem too hard in the first six months, but with the seizures it was growing increasingly stressful. Maybe if I had never complained of being bored when I was pregnant this wouldn't have happened. Fat chance!

Monday, September 15, 1980
Dr. Matthew called with the test results from the EEG. He first asked how I was, then told me that the EEG showed "no underlying seizure disorder." Most likely it had been a hypoglycemic seizure, but since there was no documentation on it he could not be positive. That was all right with me; I was sure it had to be her sugar, but would wait until it could be

documented. Again I told him I'd try to test Nancy the next time a seizure occurred, but could not make a promise. Dr. Matthew knew and accepted my feelings and my honesty. He said he understood that the testing was hard for me to do while Nancy was in the middle of a seizure, but if somehow I could manage it, the information would tell them more.

Friday, September 19, 1980
Nancy awoke with a cold. Jamie had just gotten over one, so it was not unexpected. It was her first one. I brought her to the clinic to be checked over.

Dr. Matthew examined her and said she checked out just fine. "If a fever occurs," he instructed, "use 0.6 CC of liquid Tylenol. If her temperature reaches 102°, give her a sponge bath; but if it goes any higher than that bring her in." I felt so much better just knowing she had been seen by the doctor - the basic purpose of the visit was just to reassure me that she would be all right. There would be many more of these visits in the future, I was sure. By Sunday, Nancy's cold was over.

Friday, October 3, 1980
Now Nancy had another cold, but I was not as concerned as I had been with her first. The last one had been no problem, and I felt this one would be the same. Anyway, she was cutting her teeth; mothers always claim this has a lot to do with it.

We took a ride to visit my sister-in-law Ann in North Adams, Massachusetts. She was a freshman in college this year, and lonesome. So Jamie, Nancy, my mother-in-law, and I left shortly after ten o' clock. It was a beautiful time of the year for a ride, with the foliage in full bloom. The girls snoozed on the way up, so it was quiet except for Nancy's breathing, which was loud because of her cold. When we arrived at North Adams, we found Ann and went up to her room. Or shall I say, zoo. It was a coed dorm, but it looked like a twenty-four-hour party area. There was no privacy. I guess maybe when I was seventeen I could have lived here, but of course coed dorms were not even considered then. We visited with Ann for a while, and I fed Nancy her lunch just before we left. She didn't look that well, but she did eat, so my concern was not to the point of alarm. We had previously planned to go out to lunch with Ann, but it seemed best to get Nancy home. And anyway, I was tired. I would feel more at ease with Nancy home and close to the doctors.

We stopped at McDonald's and picked up some food to go. Halfway home, I had to pull over to the side of the road. Nancy had developed diarrhea and needed immediate changing. We couldn't let that stay in the car! My mother-in-law was concerned and suggested I call the doctor when I got home. I promised her I would if Nancy didn't look any better by then. I explained to her that Nancy should be all right as long as she was eating. It was when she wouldn't eat that it was time to worry. Nancy did not look that well, but I had to consider that she did have an awful head cold. I was giving her Tylenol to help her. I tried to stay calm; I didn't want my mother-in-law to worry.

By the time we arrived home, Nancy's color was better. Mark would be home shortly, so I could ask him what I should do. Mark said she would be all right, adding that we couldn't be running to the doctor for every cold. And besides, she was eating.

I got up at midnight to feed Nancy. This was common for me, but I was feeling burnt out. Nancy was now seven months old and I was still feeding her at night. I'd cringe when I heard mothers complain that their baby was two months old and not sleeping through the night. Nancy fed poorly at midnight - it took me until after one o'clock to get her to finish the bottle. When I finally got back to bed, I barely had my eyes shut before I fell asleep.

Saturday, October 4, 1980
Mark woke me at seven to tell me that Nancy and Jamie were up. He fed Jamie and then sent her into our room to watch

television. Then he brought Nancy and laid her next to me, with the comment that she didn't look too good to him. I barely got my eyes opened to check on Nancy, but I told him I had fed her and that she didn't have to eat again until eight. I also told Mark I would call the clinic to see if someone would check her over for me.

I then asked Jamie to wake me when her cartoon show was over so I could feed Nancy.

I automatically woke up at five till eight, just like clockwork. I was still exhausted, but it was time to get up and start the day.

I picked up Nancy. She was still asleep. I carried her to the kitchen, trying to arouse her on the way, but there was no response. I grabbed her bottle and warmed it just enough to get the chill out of it. In the meantime, I rubbed sugar around her gums, again trying to arouse her. When I offered her the bottle, she wouldn't open her mouth; it was shut tight. It was eight o'clock when I picked up the phone to call for the Rescue and an ambulance. Nancy was bad- alive, yes, but whatever was going on didn't look very promising.

The EMTs in town were aware of Nancy's hypoglycemia and other health problems. Mark was an EMT, so I had no fear of who was coming to the house for us.

After I placed the call, still holding Nancy, I went downstairs to unlock the door. I climbed back upstairs to my bedroom to throw on some clothes. I put Nancy on the bed, explaining to Jamie what was happening. I told her not to worry, that someone would bring her to grandma's. All I could do was get on a pair of jeans and a shirt - there was no time for fussing at this moment.

We had a special medical alert warning system in the house, which would go off to alert all the EMTs and firemen that they had a call, and where to respond. I knew how close to the

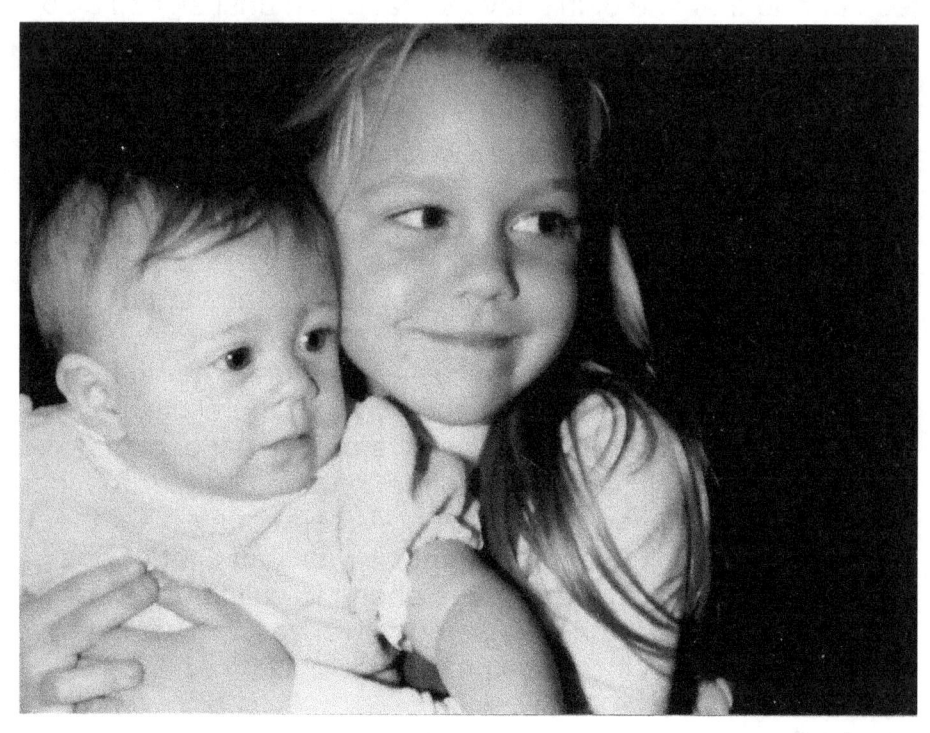

JAMIE AND NANCY

house they were, and that I didn't have much time to get ready. I quickly took Nancy and tried to feed her once more, but she wouldn't budge. I told Jamie to go in her room and find some clothes to put on while I went to the kitchen. Again I rubbed sugar on Nancy's gums.

Now the Rescue was here. I opened the back door and gave a quick sigh of relief. I explained to the fireman that Nancy refused to open her mouth to eat, so he had me sit down and hold her on my lap so he could check her out. Nancy's color was horribly pale and she was very lethargic. She was breathing, but it was very shallow and she showed no response to speak of. She did open her eyes and mouth so I could get some juice into her.

When Les, an EMT, and his friend came in, I started to cry. I was really scared now, and felt very helpless. I explained to Les that I had been trying to feed her, but that she was refusing to eat. He told me not to put the bottle in her mouth for fear she might choke. So I kept rubbing sugar around her gums and tried to explain to him what I could.

Jamie came around the corner; how my heart ached for her! When she told me she didn't know what to put on, tears came to my eyes. Just then the female EMT came in, and Les asked her to take care of Jamie. Jamie knew most of these people, so I felt secure about her, but I'm sure she was scared. I was unable to care for her just now, and I felt so badly for her. My house was a mess and I was embarrassed at myself, but there was nothing I could do but take care of Nancy.

Nancy was coming in and out. Les stayed patiently with me every minute: he was an excellent EMT and very compassionate. He calmed me down and made me feel more secure. I asked Les to call UMASS Medical to let them know I was corning in, and to have them contact Dr. Wentworth, Nancy's doctor. I then had them call Mark at work so he could meet me at the hospital.

We were now just waiting for the ambulance. I heard my front door open and a voice that was very familiar. It was my mother-in-law, crying, "Oh, no, oh no! I told you so, I told you!" Right then I quietly said to Les, "I do not need this now. Please get her out of here."
I yelled out, "She'll be fine, don't worry!"

My gosh, Nancy looked awful, but the "I told you so" was the wrong thing to say. I was furious. My father-in-law said, "Oh, boy ... did someone call Mark?" (I wanted to say "For what?") Les took over, and another EMT came out and brought my mother-in-law into the bedroom to help with Jamie.

Shortly the ambulance arrived. It was now 8:25 a.m. I brought Nancy outside, and the ambulance attendant opened the door and we got in. Nancy was taking sips of orange juice, so I held her instead of putting her on the stretcher.

As we took off, the EMT in the ambulance checked Nancy and asked me for information about what happened, medical insurance, etc. Less than halfway to the hospital, Nancy's left arm and left leg began to twitch. I told this to the EMT and asked for some sugar. There was none in the ambulance! My strength was fading. Still carrying Nancy, I followed one of the nurses to the examining room. I immediately asked the. Nurse for some Pedialyte (glucose water) so I could give it to Nancy. She brought that, and then proceeded to undress Nancy while I explained to her what was going on. I told her Nancy needed an I.V. started so we could proceed to UMASS because she was having seizures. When she undressed Nancy she said, "Oh, she hasn't even been changed yet - let me change her Pamper. "I didn't believe it; she was concerned about her wet diaper!

I then went out into the hall to check for the doctor, whom they had paged. I told a nurse that Nancy was a patient of Dr. David Matthew from the Family Health Center. A girl who was in the hall recognized his name and told me he was in the hospital. She said she would go get him. What a relief. I wouldn't be totally alone; there was someone who knew Nancy here. Then a nurse told me Mark was on the phone.

When I took the receiver, he told me that everyone was waiting for us at UMASS. I explained to him why we had stopped and reassured him that we would be there as soon as they got an I.V. started on Nancy.

The ambulance driver asked me for my insurance card as I went back to the room. I got it, and no sooner had I given it to him than the doctor they had paged entered the room. I hadn't seen any intelligent staff up to this time; I was very glad to see him. I knew I was under a lot of stress, but this nurse was way too slow. You could have dropped a bomb and I believe she would have said, "Oh my, a bomb. What shall I do?"

At any rate, I told the doctor what was going on with Nancy and that she needed an I.V. because of her hypoglycemia. It was then that I remembered I was carrying a letter from Dr. Wentworth, and gave it to him. He immediately gave the nurse orders for a blood sugar and I.V. tray. She slowly responded and he looked at her and said, "Stat!" I was happy someone was finally making her move.

The doctor then took over. He looked for a spot to start the I.V. on her head and shaved a portion of her hair. While he was starting the I.V., Dr. Matthew and Dr. Stern came in and stood beside me. I told the doctor that Dr. Matthew was Nancy's doctor and he asked Dr. Matthew if he wanted to take over. Dr. Matthew declined and turned to talk with me. With tears in my eyes, I told him how puzzled I had been to find Nancy in this condition, because I knew she had been fed as usual within the recommended eight hours. I told him I just didn't know what happened. He reassured me that I had done the right thing that it was all right. Dr. Matthew seemed to think she looked okay, and said that UMASS would take good care of her. He asked me to call him and let him know how she was doing.

The I.V. went right in. What a relief! I praised the doctor for his work. When it came to starting I.V.s, Nancy had not had an easy history.

The ambulance driver showed up and asked me how much longer we would be. I guess I hadn't realized how long we had been there, but it was obvious they did. I told him it shouldn't be much longer now that the I.V. was in. A few minutes later the doctor was all done and told me Nancy could be transferred. The blood sugar reading was now 84- her sugar level was fine now. We were then able to proceed to UMASS for further treatment.

> 10-4-80 - "Seizure Activity"
> 1st Admission
> Discharged 10-4-80

When we arrived at the UMASS Medical Center they were waiting for us. Mark met us outside and Nancy was taken into the Trauma Room. The doctor and staff immediately took over and went to work on Nancy. Dr. Mills told me he had spoken with Dr. Wentworth and had received her orders for a test on Nancy.

Then he said, "Tell me exactly what happened up till now." I explained what had taken place from the time she started her cold until we arrived at UMASS, answering all questions about my pregnancy and family history. To stop the seizures, they started Nancy on phenobarbital. Nancy was still having seizures off and on, as she had in the ambulance. She needed this medication in order to control them.

At this point, I was losing all sense of what was going on, but I kept trying to understand. Later, in the Trauma Room, Mark told me I needed a break and sent me out to the waiting room to have a coffee. I told Mark I had no idea why Nancy had ended up in this condition, since she had been eating well. I was mentally exhausted from all the questions I had had to answer within the past few hours. I just needed to clear my head.

Then Dr. Mills came into the waiting room to ask permission to give Nancy a spinal tap. My heart dropped. "Why?" I asked. Dr. Mills replied that they had ruled out just about everything that could possibly be wrong with her, and with her high temperature they would have to check for infectious meningitis. He said that she probably didn't have it, but in order to rule it out a spinal tap would be needed. Then I remembered that in August my sister Tina's little girl had come down with meningitis and almost died from it. I told Dr. Mills about it, explaining to him that Nancy had no regular contact with her because they live in New Jersey, but that they had come up recently to visit. I wanted to rule out any possibility that she had carried it to Nancy.

Dr. Mills reassured me that Tina's child could not have given meningitis to Nancy because she had received proper treatment for the meningitis and had been well for several weeks before their visit. I okayed the spinal tap, and I asked the doctor to come and get me as soon as it was finished so I could be with Nancy. I was not going to watch them do a spinal tap on Nancy; I had seen enough so far. Dr. Mills told me he should be able to tell if Nancy had meningitis as soon as he looked at the spinal fluid - if it was clear, Nancy was fine. The lab results would still be necessary to completely rule it out, but just looking at the spinal fluid would give him a good judgment on it.

So we waited. I was a nervous wreck because I knew what meningitis can do to a child. Mark kept telling me to calm down, that Nancy would be all right.

Dr. Mills returned with a smile. The fluid was clear. I'd never felt more relieved than I was to hear that, and Dr. Mills understood. I had kept in constant contact with my sister Tina while her daughter had been hospitalized with meningitis, so very ill, with death not far away. All I could do was wonder how Nancy would cope with that in addition to all her other problems. But now it was ruled out. I could put it behind me and go forward, determined not to create unnecessary problems for myself.

We spent four hours in the emergency room. Most of that time Dr. Mills was with Nancy. He diagnosed her as having a "seizure disorder" and said the test results should tell him if anything else was there.

Around 2:00 p.m. Nancy was brought up to the pediatric ICU. Mark had gone back to work and was planning to come by later to bring me home. I had thought all the questioning was over until the nurse sat down with me to go over Nancy's "normal" routine. This wasn't too bad, but I couldn't understand why they would need to know her "normal" routine when there was nothing going on with her at the moment that was normal! I knew they didn't want to bother me with all these questions, but for the hospital records and the nurses' information they had to know.

When Mark arrived shortly after four and asked if we should go home, I was ready. I had left home at 8:30 that morning; nothing had been done for myself or for my household all day, and I needed to get back there and pull my thoughts together. As we were about to leave, Dr. Mills wanted to speak with us. We asked him if we could leave now, and he gave his okay but just wanted to go back to the beginning and review what had happened to Nancy one more time. I asked him why we had to go through all this again, arguing that today alone I had already explained the situation four or five times. Dr. Mills explained that he wanted to be sure he hadn't overlooked anything. He looked as beat as I felt. I would have loved to find a place where I could go off and sleep for the next week, but that wasn't likely to happen. So once again we went over the whole thing: from relatives to pregnancy and up to seven months of age. "That's about it for now," the doctor said. As soon as we heard him say that, we said a quick, "Goodbye; you have our number!" With a smile, he said, "Yes."

It was six o'clock when we got to Mark's parents' house to pick up Jamie. They asked how Nancy was, and I answered that she was fine. I know it was hard for them to understand, but from 8:00 in the morning to 5:30 in the afternoon I had answered so many questions that I would have agreed to anything! I did tell them it had been a long day and that the testing was not fully completed. Soon we left for home and went to bed early. I made plans to go with Mark to the hospital before he went on to work so I could spend the day with Nancy.

Right around 11:30 p.m. I awoke from a sound sleep. I started to worry about Nancy and attempted to call the hospital, but fought with the fear that I might make a fool of myself. I supposed she was all right, but had a strong sense that something had happened. After awhile I managed to get back to sleep.

Sunday, October 5, 1980
Mark dropped me off at the hospital around eight-thirty. I was amazed that I was able to find my way up to the fifth floor, to the Pediatric Intensive Care Unit. The place was a zoo! It reminded me of the way Mass. General in Boston had been the time I had gone in to visit a relative of mine who had suffered a massive heart attack. It seemed just like a shopping mall at Christmas time - the corridors were as wide as a street and people were going every which way. I thought, "Someone could make a million just being a guide in this place." It may have been a marvelous hospital, but you couldn't tell who were visitors and who was staff.

When I went in to see Nancy, she looked good. The nurse had given her a bath and had washed her hair. I could tell that they made a practice of taking good care of their patients. I noticed that Nancy had a tooth showing on the bottom. I was sure this must have caused the cold she had.

Then the nurse came in and briefed me on how the night had gone. She reported that at 11:30 p.m. Nancy had suffered another seizure, but no one knew why it had happened. I thought to myself, "That's why I woke up."

Then Dr. Mills came in, and we exchanged comments on how well-rested we each looked since we had last seen one another. He told me that very little had changed with Nancy; she had undergone a seizure the night before, but her sugar levels were all right. Dr. Mills also said that her thyroid level was way up, and that he had absolutely no explanation for it. He told me that if she remained stable for the next twenty-four hours, they would transfer her to the floor tomorrow.

After everyone had left and the room had quieted down, Nancy fell asleep. I sat in the rocking chair next to her crib and began to say my prayers for her. No sooner had I begun to pray than I stopped. I wasn't sure why, but something told me just to concentrate on caring for Nancy, that prayers were already being said for her. All my energy was to be used for her. The rest of the day passed pretty quickly, and before I knew it I was back home.

Monday, October 6, 1980
Back at the hospital, I found that Nancy had done well through the night and that the doctor would have her transferred to the floor sometime that evening.

Then Dr. Wentworth came in and we talked. She told me that she could not explain the high thyroid level reading and would have to retest her. She informed me that Nancy would be placed on a daily dosage of cortisone from now on because she needed it. This was not an entirely unexpected development, and in fact Dr. Wentworth didn't know just how long Nancy would last without it. Dr. Wentworth instructed me to give her 2.5 milligrams or 1 1/2 tablet of cortisone daily, and whenever she got ill to increase the doses to twice a day. Whenever she wouldn't eat or was sick, I was to give her the cortisone. If she got worse, I was to bring her to the doctors because another increase may be needed, depending on the illness.

That evening after I had arrived home, Dr. Matthew called to ask how I was. He had seen Nancy, and told me that they were planning to do a clear urine test on her tomorrow. The procedure would involve injecting a needle into the bladder and removing the urine. Yuck! I was glad he told me, because nothing had been mentioned to me about it. Dr. Matthew also let me know he would be at UMASS around 1:30 p.m. tomorrow and asked if I would be there. I told him I would.

Tuesday, October 7, 1980
I left for the hospital around noontime. When I arrived, I found that Nancy had been transferred to the floor. She was in a large room with three other patients. One child, about a year old, was in a cast up to her waist. The nurse told me she had had an operation and would be wearing it for several weeks. The child had to remain on her stomach the whole time she would be in the cast. The only time she could change positions was when her mother came in to hold her. It was interesting to see her mother holding her - I'm sure the child weighed fifty pounds or more with the cast.

The child next to her was in a croup tent. Then there was Johnny, next to Nancy. Johnny was mentally retarded and had cerebral palsy, a multiple handicap. He was a permanent resident of the hospital. They kept him on a respirator and only fed him bland food, which he would drink through a straw while the nurse held it.

Around one o' clock, Dr. Kim came in to draw urine from Nancy. I told him I knew this was necessary, but asked why it hadn't been done sooner. He didn't know why, but said the urine had to be drawn after a feeding to be sure there was urine in her bladder. He left, returning with a syringe and some other material. As Dr. Kim got Nancy ready, I was patiently waiting for a nurse to show up so I could leave. All of a sudden he asked me to hold Nancy for him. I was shocked to find myself doing it! Dr. Kim cleansed the bladder area, below the stomach, and just before injecting the needle he said, "I hope she has some in there." My God, I thought, he better pray there is or I'll be screaming at him along with Nancy! As he injected the needle, she screamed. I could feel the pain myself and was ready to cry. This needle was large, not just the kind they use to give a regular shot. But bingo! Urine was there and in a few seconds it was over. Dr. Kim left to get it to the lab for testing, and I - in a state of shock - held Nancy. I told her it was all right, and that I was sorry. I couldn't believe the doctor had done this procedure without a nurse. I guess he had a lot of faith in me. My impression of him was not the greatest; he had not shown any emotion toward either me or Nancy. I was totally amazed.

Dr. Matthew came in at 1:30 p.m. and made a funny comment about Nancy's hairstyle. There was much more hair gone, right where it had already grown in once from the shaving done for her previous I.V.s. After checking Nancy over, he told me she looked good. He informed me that she had a urinary tract infection, and I exclaimed, "What?" No one had told me anything about that. Nancy had been through all this just because of a bladder infection? Then Dr. Matthew explained that this was the reason they had taken the urine sample directly from the bladder – to make sure it was correct. (I remembered the conversation I had with my mother the evening after the test had been done. She had guessed that they had put a catheter on Nancy, and as a result she was infected. Sure enough, it was true; whatever problems she had been admitted with, she would be leaving with more.)

Dr. Matthew talked with me awhile, explaining what was going on. I told him how Dr. Kim had done the test with me assisting him, and I asked Dr. Matthew why there had not been a nurse there. He replied that he didn't know why it had happened that way, but said that I should not have been made to do it. I guess I wasn't forced to assist him, but I had simply bowed to his expectation.

Wednesday, October 8, 1980
It was now definite that Nancy had a urinary tract infection.

They had put her on medication for it, and she was expected to be released on Friday.

Thursday, October 9, 1980
Today Dr. Kim came in to ask me if I could do a short interview on camera with him for an assignment he'd been given. I advised him that I needed to leave in twenty minutes, but he assured me we would be done in time.

Dr. Kim and I hurried downstairs and finally found the place he had set up for the interview. I was laughing; even a fourth year medical student who worked here was lost! The interview turned out to be fun - I enjoyed it and laughed through most of it. He questioned me about how I had taken the news of Nancy's disease. I answered that I did not consider her condition to be a disease, because to me a disease was something that ate away at you, and Nancy's problem was not like that. I called it a disorder or a malfunction, because there was simply a part of her that was not working properly. He laughed at the word "malfunction." I told him it was like a car that wasn't working right -you have to make a replacement in order for it to run properly. He asked several questions, mostly about my family and how Nancy had changed my life. I was done in time to get Mark to work and myself home.

Friday, October 10, 1980
Now it was time for us to go to the hospital to pick up Nancy. Jamie was happy about it; she hadn't seen Nancy for almost a week and really missed her. Shortly after we arrived, Dr.Wentworth came to give Nancy a prerelease checkup. We went over her medications and when to give her the cortisone. Then we were on our way home.

It felt good bringing Nancy home - it had been a long week. I was given a prescription for a ten-day supply of ampicillin to treat Nancy's urinary tract infection, and then I was told to make a follow-up appointment with Dr. Matthew. I had already called Dr. Matthew earlier to let him know Nancy was being discharged and would be in on Thursday for a well-child checkup. I appreciated the good communication between Dr. Matthew and myself. I kept him well informed on everything that was happening to Nancy.

The week I had spent with Nancy in that hospital room, watching the other children on the floor, made me conclude that my child had the easiest type of disability to live with. It seemed that no matter what your child was up against, there was always someone worse off.. like Johnny -although he may have been happy in his own way.

Thursday, October 16, 1980
At 11 :00 a.m. I brought Nancy to see Dr. Matthew for her well-child checkup. She weighed in at 14 lbs., 10 oz., and measured 24 3/4 inches long. My record for this day reads: "She was sitting up with some support, but fell when there was none. Most everything else was up to the seven-month level. It was taken into consideration that she had been in the hospital." Dr. Matthew and I went over the cortisone levels to be given when Nancy was ill. The record again reads: "For any fever greater than 102°or if she will not eat, increase cortisone 2.5 mg. 2 times per day. If no sign of improvement, I am to bring her in." Dr. Matthew asked me to bring in a sample of Nancy's urine tomorrow so it could be tested. The nurse then gave me a pediatric bag to put on Nancy so I could collect the urine. It was fairly simple to do; I had seen the nurses do it frequently, so instructions were not needed.

Friday, October 17, 1980
I looked forward to having my mother come after work tonight to stay over and visit with the girls, and especially with me. The whole time Nancy had been in the hospital, my family had kept in close touch. If I wasn't at the hospital, I would be talking on the phone. It was disruptive to my immediate family life, and it felt as though I had been up around the clock for a week, but I had managed. The support from my family had been the best part.

When I spoke to our friend Tom's wife, Lisa, she told me that she had requested prayers for Nancy at the Sunday service on the 5th of this month. I then questioned her to find out the exact time she had requested the prayers. Puzzled, she replied, "After ten o'clock." Then I told her about how I had been sitting with Nancy in the hospital that morning and had tried to begin praying when I was "told" not to. I didn't hear a voice or anything, but a strong feeling had come over me - a sense that I should stop and save my energy for Nancy's care. Now I knew why: Lisa and the whole church were already praying. I thanked her very much.

Saturday, October 25, 1980
This was the most important day yet for me with Nancy - she said "Mama" for the first time! I celebrated all day long, and everyone I spoke to heard all about it. I'm sure Mark and Jamie were tired of it all by the end of the day, but~ knew I deserved every minute of it.

Tuesday, October 28, 1980
Yesterday Nancy turned seven months old, and today she saw snow for the first time. There was just a little, but winter was on its way. Nancy had a morning appointment with Dr. Wentworth at the clinic at UMASS. Because all Dr. Wentworth needed was to draw blood for a repeated thyroid test, I would be able to come in anytime during the morning.

NOVEMBER 1980

Monday, November 17, 1980
Nancy went for a well-child checkup with Dr. Matthew today. She had her DPT shot and was scheduled to come back in three weeks for her OPV. Nancy was doing well, with no illnesses.

This particular day it was snowing, and it continued until the next day. By the time the storm stopped on Tuesday we had eight inches on the ground. I had always enjoyed the snow, but since having Nancy, snowstorms were making me nervous. There was always the concern that yet another medical crisis would erupt during a storm, making it impossible to get her to a doctor or hospital. I might be left in a helpless panic, not knowing what to do.

Tuesday November 18, 1980
Dr. Wentworth called with instructions to increase Nancy's synthroid (her thyroid replacement) medication to 35 micrograms per day. She explained that it was a safe increase, since 35 micro. was still fairly low. She would plan to see Nancy next week.

I promptly called Dr. Matthew to let him know that her medication level had changed. Keeping up with Nancy's treatment changes was not too difficult, since I was always one to handle such things right away. Anytime her medication was changed, I had to inform each of her doctors as soon as possible so they could update their records. It was crucial not to delay these communications, because in the event of an emergency the records would show an accurate account. I shuddered at any prospect of my having to recall all her prescriptions under that kind of pressure!

Tuesday November 25, 1980
Nancy had her well-child checkup with Dr. Wentworth at 11 :30 this morning. It was mainly just to keep a close watch on her. Thankfully no blood was necessary, so we got through quickly.

DECEMBER 1980

Monday, December 8, 1980
During Nancy's well-child checkup with Dr. Matthew today, we found that she now weighed 16 lbs. 10 oz. and was 26 1/4 inches long. Nancy had begun to sit up without support and had reached the level of an eight-month-old. She took her OPV drink, and was rescheduled to see Dr.Matthew again in two months.

Thursday, December 11, 1980
I discovered that Nancy had come down with a cold. She was

acting the way she did when she was hypoglycemic. She was attentive and playing normally, but I called Dr. Matthew, wanting to know if I should increase her cortisone as I had been instructed to do by Dr. Wentworth. He promised he would get back to me shortly about it.

When I talked with Dr. Matthew again, he said he had spoken with Dr. Wentworth, who had advised not to increase the cortisone. When I explained that Nancy was having a hard time breathing when drinking her bottle, Dr. Matthew prescribed 1/2 teaspoon of Dimetapp, twice daily. This would help dry up her nasal passage so she could drink her bottle normally. I questioned Dr. Matthew about why Dr. Wentworth advised against increasing her cortisone, since I was told last October that I was to increase it when she became ill. He pointed out that the cortisone would stunt Nancy's growth; the less of it she had at this time the more she would grow. Okay, I would do as I was told. Part of me felt all right about this decision, but naturally I was concerned about the effect of this cold, and every cold thereafter. Dr. Matthew asked me to call if I needed him, and told me to stop the Dimetapp as soon as Nancy was eating well.

Thursday, December 18, 1980
At 6:30 a.m., Nancy suffered another seizure. I fed her orange juice with extra sugar added, and rubbed liquid sugar on her gums. The liquid sugar was from decorative cake jell that I had purchased ahead of time with this purpose in mind. Dr. Wentworth had given me the tip that this was the quickest way to get the sugar into her. She ate extremely well, and within ten minutes she became perfectly alert. My nerves had exhausted me, but I knew that as long as she was responding to me she would be all right for now.

I called the clinic at eight-thirty. They told me to bring Nancy in at 10:15 a.m. to see Dr. Matthew.

When we arrived, the first thing Dr. Matthew did was to calm me down. It was quite evident to him that at the moment, I needed more help than Nancy did. Then he had a blood test done on her, and checked her reflexes and vision. He remarked that she seemed fine, and most likely had undergone a hypoglycemic seizure. It was still not officially documented that the cause of Nancy's seizures was hypoglycemia, even though the evidence had led us to believe it was. As he had told me earlier, a specific test would be needed. Nancy drank down 6 1/2 ounces of formula while Dr. Matthew went to check on the results of the blood test. When he returned, he told me that her level was low, only 37. However, since Nancy was eating, the chance of another seizure at this point was slim. I was to feed her more frequently; then she should be all right.

Sunday, December 21, 1980
Today we held a special Christmas celebration at my father's house. Since all of us had our own families now, we had agreed to get everyone together the Sunday before Christmas so we wouldn't miss each other.

While we were at my Dad's, Nancy took a nap and slept for quite awhile. I realized that she had been sleeping too long. It was nearly time for her to eat. When I went to get her, she really did not want to wake up. She was lethargic and covered with sweat. Not wanting to cause a scene, I settled myself on the couch, where it was quiet, and gave her a bottle. She was drinking down her formula like crazy. I knew the signs that her sugar was low, but sat praying that she would be all right. It wasn't that I was afraid to let my family know; it was just that we were all celebrating Christmas and everyone was having such a good time. I hated to spoil it, and thankfully I didn't have to. After her feeding, Nancy was fine.

Monday, December 22, 1980
Nancy was not eating well. I called the clinic, and Dr. Matthew told me to bring her in for a fasting blood sugar test. I went straight to the clinic lab, where the test results showed her blood sugar to be extremely low - only 22! Dr. Matthew instructed me to start feeding her at four in the morning. From

now on, she was not to go more than five hours without feeding. "Go in for FBS when the cold is over," he said. "Phenob. level was 18.5."

Thursday, December 25, 1980
The next two days were filled with celebration, especially because it was Nancy's first Christmas. We held our traditional Christmas Eve celebration at my in-laws' house. Then on Christmas Day we went back to their place, as always, to exchange gifts in the afternoon.

Friday, December 26, 1980
It was comforting to have Dr. Matthew call to see how we were doing. He asked me to come in on Monday so he could test Nancy's blood sugar. He also let me know that he would be on vacation the next week, but that there would be a resident at the clinic in case I needed someone.

That was okay with me; at least I knew ahead of time. I told him that Dr. Wentworth would also be gone that week, so it would be up to me to treat Nancy on my own for the first time. Dr. Matthew reassured me that the resident knew about Nancy, and that he had left explicit instructions regarding her treatment.

Saturday, December 27, 1980
Nancy was nine months old today. She awoke with a stuffy nose - another cold. Even so, today was a special day: a priest with a healing ministry was coming to the Congregational church in town to conduct a healing service at 12: 15 p.m. The church had put aside a ticket so we could come. The only hitch was that I was nervous about taking her now that she wasn't feeling well.

My mother called, and I told her Nancy was all stuffed up. She urged me to go anyway, and not to let Satan keep me away. As she encouraged me, I saw that it was exactly Satan's purpose to try to keep me away from a divine healing service. I thanked my mom for helping me see things in their true light.

It was important for me to take Nancy; I just didn't want her to be sick.

Then I called Lisa, Tom's wife. She had been praying for Nancy, and was the one who had secured my ticket. I let her know that Nancy was feeling sick, but that I was still going to go. It would be easier to stay home, I told her, but Satan wasn't going to keep me here no matter what obstacles came in the way. Nancy was going to be blessed by the priest today and make it through the service.

Jamie would be staying with my mother-in-law for the afternoon. She really wanted to go with me, but I knew I could not handle a four-year-old in addition to Nancy for the afternoon at a church service.

The church was located only a quarter of a mile from my house. We arrived there at 11:45 a.m., a half-hour ahead of time. I had procured tickets for two friends of mine, and we all sat together in the back row. One of these women was suffering from muscular dystrophy, although she was able to walk and function with it. It was a joy for her to be there.

The service began at 12:15 p.m. as planned, and proved to be a very moving experience. Throughout the afternoon, the church building was so filled with the Holy Spirit that it felt like heaven. During the service I kept a close watch on Nancy. I had hoped the priest would come to her separately to bless her, but it was still okay even when he didn't.

I fed Nancy juice while the service was in progress, and no sooner was she finished than she vomited all over me. Great. Now what do I do? I left the service and went downstairs to get us both cleaned up. I was upset with myself. Nancy had been fine; I had simply overfed her. When we were presentable, I headed back up the stairs for the rest of the service. I could feel weariness from sitting all afternoon, and just from the wonder of being present in a place where there was so much open praise for the Lord. It was wonderful. I had never been to a healing service before, nor had I ever seen people with such open praise for God. My religious training had never included such things; it was deeply moving.

At around four o'clock, the priest announced that those who would like to be blessed, or to have him lay hands on them, could come forward to the front of the church. The minister of the Congregational church motioned for me to come forward and get in line with Nancy. As soon as I rose to go, holding Nancy, tears welled up in my eyes. I watched intently as the people who were ahead of me in line received prayer. Some fell to the floor, with helpers standing ready behind them so they would not be injured. I had a fleeting concern that I might fall while holding Nancy, but comforted myself with the realization that God would not allow her to be harmed.

Our time was here; I was next. The priest looked at me and asked, "What is Wrong with your child?" I told him she had a rare illness and that more testing would have to be done. Then I began to cry. The priest took Nancy from me, lifted her up in his hands and prayed for her. He gave her back to me, and I felt myself sway backward a little. He then placed his hands on my head and prayed over me. After his hands left my head, I again felt myself swaying back. I said "Thank you" and returned to my seat. I had been "slain in the Spirit" twice - once for myself and once for Nancy. I felt great relief. Now all I could do was to wait for the testing to be done.

At some point, major testing on Nancy's growth pattern was going to take place, and I was just going to wait and see what the results would be. I believed what I had been told - that a healing takes place in God's time, not always immediately. But pinpointing the time that Nancy would be tested gave me something to look forward to. For awhile I searched intently for signs of change, but soon put it out of my way and just waited for God to decide the best time.

Sunday, December 28, 1980
I fed Nancy once at 3:00 a.m. and then woke her up again at

eight o'clock to give her breakfast. She was hypoglycemic again - a fairly light seizure compared to the others, but another just the same. At around nine, Nancy vomited. She was still congested, so I called the clinic and spoke with Dr. Lynn. I explained what was going on and told her that I wanted to increase Nancy's daily dosage to 2.5 mg. of cortisone twice a day, instead of just once. I needed to check with a doctor to be sure it was all right. After looking up Nancy's chart, she agreed with me. She said she would see me the next morning when I brought Nancy in for her fasting blood sugar test.

Monday, December 29, 1980
Eight-thirty found me at the clinic with Nancy for her five-hour fasting blood sugar testing. Her level was up to 70! At nine o'clock Dr. Lynn took a look at her. After examining her, the doctor said there was some minor congestion, but nothing severe. She had another doctor come in to listen to Nancy's chest, and he agreed with Dr. Lynn.

It was not unusual for one of the staff doctors to be called in to give a second opinion, especially in Nancy's case. Here at the clinic, the residents were medical doctors who were doing their residency in family medicine. It gave them experience with families and prepared them for their own future practices.

Dr. Lynn felt Nancy would be all right, and instructed me to decrease the cortisone back to her daily dosage of 2.5 mg.

"College of Hard Knocks"

Tuesday, December 30, 1980
At 12:30 in the afternoon, as I was preparing Nancy's lunch, I noticed her eyes blinking rapidly. I quickly gave her a bottle, talking to her the whole time and reassuring her that she would be all right. To myself, I kept reciting the Lord's prayer to give me strength. Nancy came around quickly and seemed to be acting normally.
I put in another call to the clinic, which Dr. Lynn shortly returned. I told her I was now comfortable with Nancy, but

wanted to report that she had another seizure - this time during the day, which was unusual. Dr. Lynn told me she would be at the clinic the rest of the day if I needed her.

It was around 4:00 p.m. that I noticed Nancy sweating- another sign. That was it, as far as I was concerned. She had eaten at twelve-thirty and now, only four hours later, she was showing signs again. I was worried now. I called the clinic and asked the doctor if she would see Nancy. Mark was working, so my mother-in-law drove me to the clinic. Jamie stayed with her aunt.

We arrived at the clinic around five p.m. Dr. Lynn took Nancy right to the emergency room to draw blood. She checked her phenobarbital level and took a sugar reading at the same time. Nancy's sugar level was 70. She vomited twice while we were there; she was still congested and crying hard from the blood testing. Dr. Lynn decided to start an I.V.

The doctor then told me that she was going to increase Nancy's phenobarbital and admit her to the hospital for observation overnight. That was fine with me; home was not the place for Nancy tonight. "Will she be able to go home in the morning?" I asked. Most likely, the doctor responded.

Back in the waiting room, I explained to my mother-in-law that Nancy was headed for the hospital overnight and that I would be staying with her. This was no surprise to her, since she just spent quite awhile listening to Nancy's crying and had readily assumed that Nancy would be admitted. Since the I.V. had already been started, Nancy would be going by ambulance. There was nothing further my mother-in-law could do, so I sent her home.

The ambulance arrived, and Nancy and I were off to UMASS Medical.

> 6:00 p.m. **"12-30-80 Admission to UMASS Medical
> Seizure disorder
> Discharged 12-31-80"

When we arrived at UMASS, we were brought into the Trauma room. I met with the doctor and nurse, updating them on Nancy's history from birth to the present. I was getting pretty good at answering their questions; the answers were always the same. The first thing they did was to increase her phenobarbital to 50 mg. to halt the seizure activity.

As soon as he could, Mark came down from work to check on us and see what was happening. He wasn't very happy when I told him of my decision to stay the night with Nancy in the hospital.

Since she would be discharged in the morning, it was easier for me to stay rather than leave at midnight and try to get back there first thing in the morning. Mark's parents would pick us up when Nancy was ready to be released. Mark stayed for about an hour then, returned to work.

I had informed the nurse that Nancy was due to eat at five o'clock and that I would like to give her a bottle if I could. I had none with me. The nurse replied that Nancy was getting enough nourishment from the I.V, but said I could try.

Well, it was very busy in there with three other patients, and before I knew it one thing had led to another and it was seven-thirty. Now Nancy was getting cranky. I tried to calm her down, and again stated to the nurse that Nancy may be hungry. I didn't dare ask the second time for a bottle; she hadn't given me one the first time and I was afraid of her reaction if I bothered her again about it. Although I knew Nancy better than anyone else there, I had the sinking feeling that if I demanded too much or showed knowledge above theirs I would somehow be in trouble. It was a tense situation: this was Nancy's second admission and her doctor was out of town. The doctor who was to care for Nancy was a neurologist, Dr. Adams, who had only seen her briefly. But they had to put someone down on paper, and neither of Nancy's own doctors were around. I could not leave Nancy alone.

Finally Nancy fell asleep. I had forgotten again about the need for her to eat. When Nancy began to sweat at 8:30 p.m., I called for the nurse. She looked at how wet the hair was, and pronounced that it must be the medication. I gave the nurse a puzzled look. "She hasn't eaten since twelve-thirty. Don't you think it ' s a sign of hypoglycemia?" I asked. The nurse said, "No-they gave her 50 mg. of phenobarbital., and I think they gave her too much." Again, I felt I'd better be quiet. The last thing I needed was to have the nurse mad at me. I didn't want to be that "hysterical" mother!

After the nurse went off I touched Nancy. She was clammy. I checked her eyes, and they were wandering. I then felt her mouth to see if her bite was rigid. It was. I knew then that she was having a seizure, and that I would have to take my stand no matter what. I was going to give the orders now! I called to the nurse to get a doctor, informing her that Nancy was having a seizure. To my amazement, she actually listened! (She had to-I meant business.) "Get me some milk," I said with authority. Before I knew it, two female doctors rushed in. One looked quickly at Nancy and immediately called for a blood sugar and glucose. She administered the glucose I.V. while the other doctor checked Nancy more thoroughly. During all this, another nurse ran in and handed me the milk I had asked for - in a carton! What I needed was a bottle; anyone knew a nine-month-old couldn't drink out of a carton! She ran off to get the bottle. Then the second doctor ordered a chest X-ray. I looked her in the eye and demanded, "Why?" She explained that she heard "crackling" and needed a chest X-ray to determine if there was pneumonia. I snapped, "She doesn't. She's in here for a phenobarbital increase; can't it wait?"

The look on the doctor's face was remarkable: utter shock. "Several doctors have listened to her chest over the past two days," I went on,"- four just today. No one felt she may have pneumonia. Can it wait until morning?" The doctor countered, "Well, I would really like an X-ray." "Is this necessary?" I demanded. "Well!" she huffed. "I'll allow an X-ray in the morning if you feel it's necessary, but not until then," I shot back. "Nancy is having a seizure -that's all!" The doctor left-upset, I'm sure - and I never saw her again.

The nurse came back with the bottle of milk, which Nancy drank down in record time. The nurse made no apology for her mistake. Then the nurse from the ER came over to me, saying, "It's about time!" "What?" I asked. She explained that I was one of the first mothers she had ever heard telling a doctor "no" on an X-ray. "They love to take X-rays around here!" she remarked. I replied that it may be true, but that Nancy was in here explicitly for an increase in medication; and that was all she was going to be treated for unless someone could prove me wrong . When the results of the blood sugar test came back, the level was all the way down to 18. That spoke for itself.

For the first time in nine months, I was in charge! They were listening to me, and it felt good. I allowed them to do their job; they were the experts up to this point. But I had no Dr. Matthew or Dr. Wentworth to take over. They were on vacation, and I was in control. After all, I was the only one around who knew Nancy. I didn't like myself for having to be pushed to this limit, but they had given me no choice. They simply would not listen. I had to be Nancy's voice; my little girl could only show me familiar signs that she needed help. At times I carried guilty feelings that I didn't sense Nancy's needs soon enough, but it was hard for me, too. I was giving Nancy all my love and protection. I knew we had a bond, and that she was with me all the way. It took a lot of patience from both of us.

It was ten-thirty when they brought Nancy up to the pediatric floor. The nurses on the floor went to get me a bed so I could stay beside Nancy for the night. The resident on duty on that floor came in to introduce herself as Dr. Ryan. We spoke briefly. I told her that Nancy would need a feeding at 12:30 a.m., and that I would be willing to feed her. I also made it

82

known that I did not want what had happened downstairs to be repeated, and she agreed. Dr. Ryan let me know that she would not be back in and urged me to be sure I told the night nurse, who would be in shortly. I glanced at Dr. Ryan's name tag. "Family Practice," it read. No wonder I liked her.

The nurse on the eleven-to-seven shift got in shortly after 11:30 p.m. I requested a bottle of milk (I stressed the word bottle!) for 12:30 a.m. to give Nancy. She was about to go on rounds, but would be done by then and promised to bring one .in to me.

Wednesday, December 31, 1980
My plan was to stay up until 12:30, then get some sleep after Nancy had been fed. I watched the clock and waited. Twelve-thirty went by, but no bottle came. I waited some more. Nancy seemed all right, and I knew she certainly wasn't the only patient on the floor. At 1 :00 a.m., I took a walk to the lounge as a good excuse to find out where the nurse might be. As I passed the nurses' station, there she sat, doing paperwork. By now I was ticked, but I kept on toward the lounge, gathering my feelings under control. If I hadn't passed by her, I probably would have lost my cool, but I had too much pride to lower myself to her level. Five or ten minutes went by, and as I headed back to Nancy's room, I stopped at the nurses' station. The night nurse just sat there, ignoring me. She knew I was there, but she was going to let me stand there until she was good and ready to look up.

When she finally did look up, I asked her if I could have a bottle for Nancy so I could feed her. "Nancy was to have eaten at 12:30 a.m.," I chided gently. "Sure," she replied, 'I'll bring it down for you." I thanked her and returned to Nancy's room. I waited. A few times I heard footsteps in the corridor, but no one entered the room. I had no idea what time it was, but I knew she still wasn't coming. My patience had hit the limit. When I got back to the nurses ' station, the clock on the wall read 2:00 a.m.! The nurse was still at her paperwork!

I spotted another nurse, who asked if she could be of help. I explained wearily that Nancy had been due for her bottle at 12:30 a.m., and that I would like to feed her so I could get some rest. She asked, "Who's her nurse?" and checked on the board to find out. Then she realized it was the girl behind the desk. She addressed the girl, demanding to know why Nancy's bottle had still not been brought to me. "I've been doing paperwork," she said. The head nurse then ordered her to get Nancy's mother a bottle and to forget her paperwork. The head nurse was not happy about the situation, and I shared her feeling. I told the head nurse I would have prepared the bottle myself if I had known where to find it. She let me know she was sorry, and that there was no excuse for this.

It took the nurse less than a minute - no exaggeration - to get the bottle and give it to me. I did thank her, but I made a mental note to inform Dr. Wentworth of her behavior. I couldn't believe what was happening; she was the first nurse who had ever given me this kind of problem. I didn't even know her from a previous admittance. She belonged behind a desk, all right, but she had the wrong profession!

I was awakened around four when the nurse came in. I noted wryly to myself that this was the first time this nurse had set foot in here since I had seen her go off duty at 11:30 the morning before! Nancy and I were on our way home by 11 o'clock. Her phenobarbital had been increased to 15 mg. in the morning, and 30 mg at night. She would be checked by her family physician on Friday as a follow-up.

I spoke with Dr. Wentworth soon after she returned from her vacation. She had called me about Nancy's admission. I reported the incident with the night nurse to her, only because it was so important that Nancy ate on time. Dr. Wentworth was very disturbed by it and thanked me for letting her know. She then confided that they had been having quite a bit of trouble with incidents of diabetics not being fed on time on that particular floor. I told her that I realized there are other patients and would not complain if the nurse had been busy with someone else, but added that in this case the nurse had been out of line. Dr. Wentworth agreed that there was no excuse whatsoever for what had occurred, assuring me that she intended to make sure it did not happen again. I gave her the name of the nurse· responsible so that the conscientious ones would not be unfairly reprimanded.

Until this incident, I had always praised the nursing staff, who often over worked during their eight hours. But in this case, I felt it my duty to complain -- only to protect the other patients from this nurse 's negligence.

JANUARY 1981

Friday, January 2, 1981
This was the day for Nancy's follow-up check by Dr. Matthew. She weighed in at 17 lbs. 12 oz. It was a relief to know that she hadn't lost any weight from her hospital stay. Dr. Matthew and I discussed her admission. He told me that her blood sugar reading in the hospital was down to 18. I already knew this, but he was glad because this was the first reading ever taken while she was actually in the middle of a seizure. Now they had documentation, which supported his view that her seizures were most likely from hypoglycemia. There would be more evidence needed to prove that all of the seizures were based on low blood sugar, but they could be confident that at least this one had been.

He observed that Nancy was wheezing, and determined she had a mild bronchitis. I was to provide humidity at home, as well as nasal suction. He asked me to call him if her respiratory condition worsened, because in that case he might have to start Nancy on sylophillin. In addition, he wanted her to return in a week for a fasting blood sugar test. Nancy's cortisone was decreased to 2.5 mg., her maintenance dosage.

Friday, January 9, 1981
I took Nancy to the clinic again for her fasting blood sugar test.

After an eight hour fast, her blood sugar read 32 - too low. When Nancy was healthy, I was to feed her every seven hours. At her present age, the blood sugar level showed little sign of improvement.

I reported to Dr. Matthew that Dr. Wentworth had hopes that the growth hormone might help to boost Nancy's blood sugars. But the hypoglycemia was not enough reason to start her on growth hormone yet; she would need to have major testing done. It would be a long process, Dr. Matthew said, and could not be done while she was on increased cortisone. It could only be performed while she was free of illness. The tests, which would determine Nancy's need for growth hormone, involved a series of blood tests to be done over a full eight-hour period. During this process, she could not be allowed to eat. The test results would determine how much growth hormone, if any, Nancy's system was producing. Following the test, Dr. Wentworth would have to write up a protocol to prove Nancy's need for Human Growth Hormone.

The Growth Hormone is supplied by the Federal government. In order to receive it, Nancy would have to be accepted and approved at higher governmental levels. Obtaining government approval would involve a lot of paperwork and testing by Dr. Wentworth. It would take approximately one-and-a-half months to determine her levels and start the protocol, so the sooner she could be tested, the sooner she could be accepted into the program.

I was determined to keep Nancy healthy so she could have the testing done in the immediate future. This was my job, the goal I was aiming for. I knew I could be stubborn, and I was going to set my mind on getting this testing done. I would keep a positive attitude and look straight ahead. All I was waiting for now was a call from Dr. Wentworth, letting me know when to bring Nancy in to get started.

Monday, January 12, 1981
Nancy wouldn't take any solid food and she was also

constipated. I called the clinic and spoke with Dr. Matthew. He instructed me to give her "Senokot" - 1/4 teaspoon once a day, and to call in the morning if she still wasn't accepting any solids. He advised no increase of cortisone at this time.

Nancy didn't improve much over the next two days, but at least she was eating a few solids. Although feeding Nancy around the clock was tiring me out, I didn't feel it was necessary to bring her to the doctor again right away. Nancy was eating - not as much as I would have liked – but at least she didn't seem any worse. I was faithfully doing everything I had been told to do to relieve her wheezing and constipation.

Thursday, January 15, 1981
I awoke in time for seven o'clock and discovered Nancy in the middle of another seizure. Again I fed her sugared orange juice and rubbed liquid sugar around her gums. I noticed that Nancy's right side was twitching. It had started with her leg and then to her arm. Alarmed, I went to the bedroom to wake up Mark - mostly for support and reassurance that she would somehow be all right. Nancy was tense and cold, but after she took in four ounces of juice the twitching slowed down. She finished six ounces and began to move around. She was gaining alertness and beginning to notice Mark and me. What a relief!

I called the clinic at nine o'clock and they gave me a 2:30 p.m. appointment with Dr. Matthew. I was beginning to feel that the clinic was my second home. I was also feeling I must be a pain in the neck to the staff. I had either called or visited the clinic more than ten times in the last three weeks. I could feel shame creeping over me - the shame of being a mother who was not capable of taking care of her own daughter. Part of me knew I was doing all I could for her, but doubts about my own ability would sneak over me, leaving me bearing a vague load of guilt. At times I felt helpless, ready to give up. If the staff had asked me to leave Nancy with them I would have, without second thought. I simply failed to understand what was going on with her; I was doing everything they told me to

do and still nothing was making a difference.
When we arrived at the clinic for the 2:30 appointment, I told
Dr. Matthew what was going on:

> "Seizures 3 hours after meal, refusing solids -- formula
> only - constipated bloated stomach, asthma.
> Start theophylline - this probably causing air
> swallowing! worsening bloatedness – eating.
>
> Medications being given at this time:
> Senokot - 1/4 tsp. 2x per day/ liquid
> Elixicon - 112 tsp. 3x per day I liquid
> Mylicon drops - 4 drops 4x per day liquid

Dr. Matthew wanted me to ring the clinic on Saturday to report
how Nancy was doing to the doctor on call. He promised to
leave word so the doctor would be expecting my call. He also
reassured me that Nancy would be all right, inviting me to call
anytime I needed to. He said he would phone me tomorrow to
check on Nancy.

I felt much better. I always did after Dr. Matthew had seen
Nancy and had a talk with me. That's what was so great about
him - he talked to me, not at me. He gave me strength and
confidence when I was ready to give up. No matter how much
of a failure I felt, he had a way of turning my failure into
positive thinking. He was more than just a doctor-he was a
friend.

Friday, January 16, 1981
Dr. Matthew called me after lunch to see how we were. I
related to him that Nancy had vomited this morning, but that I
felt it was simply due to overfeeding. I promised that I would
try to get her on a better schedule. I had suffered some
moments of concern, but now I felt comfortable. Again, he
reminded me to call the clinic tomorrow and speak with the
doctor on call.

Nancy went in for her nap after lunch. Because of her labored breathing and her stuffy sinuses, I had been watching her carefully all morning. Around three o'clock I started getting nervous. She was sleeping too long, I thought. I had had her on a schedule of more frequent feedings, since she wasn't eating enough solids. Given her increased number of seizures lately, I wasn't going to let her go too long between feedings.

When I woke her, it was plain she was all stuffed up and suffering an awful head cold. I mentioned to Mark that she didn't look too well. He suggested that perhaps after she had been awake for a while she would clear up, and suggested that I simply keep an eye on her. Around three-thirty I sat down with Nancy to give her some juice. The bottle had only been in her mouth a few seconds when she suddenly stopped breathing completely and turned blue!

I yelled for Mark to come quick, screaming that she was turning blue. Panic utterly paralyzed me. Mark was at my side in seconds. He lifted Nancy from me, turned her over, and hit her on the back. She coughed up some phlegm and started to breath again. Her breathing was very shallow, so we decided it was "back to the clinic:" I called the clinic to tell them we were bringing Nancy in and asked them to inform Dr. Matthew. They told me Dr. Matthew had just left, but that Dr. Lynn would see her.

We all piled into the car and headed for the clinic. Mark was as concerned as I was, and we watched Nancy carefully all the way. She was pale and her breathing was shallow. Mark advised me to stay as calm as possible and to speak to her gently. We arrived at the clinic at 4:00 p.m. and were ushered straight to the emergency room.

Dr. Lynn and Dr. Willis entered the emergency room together. Dr. Lynn checked Nancy over and ordered that a blood sugar test be done on her. Dr. Willis asked me what had happened. But I couldn't speak through my tears; Mark had to tell him.

After I had calmed down, Dr. Willis assured me that Nancy

would be all right, adding that it shouldn't happen again. I told him that if it hadn't been for Mark I didn't know what would have happened. Mark had saved her just in time. If I had been alone with Nancy, perhaps I would have done just what Mark had known to do - but just then I doubted it.

Dr. Lynn then informed us that Nancy's blood sugar was reading at 42, which was all right. She recognized that Nancy was quite congested, but told us that the phlegm was moving and that keeping her on liquids would prevent it from building up. After we had reviewed her medications, I promised to do my best to use her bottle feedings to get all the medicine into her. Not only was Nancy on synthroid and cortisone (which I had not yet given to her that day), she was also on three other medications which Dr. Matthew had prescribed yesterday.

Dr. Lynn's instructions included feeding Nancy every three hours with five ounces of a glucose apple juice mixture. She suggested that Mark and I take turns handling her feeding shift. (I knew, however, that I was going to be the one doing these feedings.) When I asked the doctor about increasing Nancy's cortisone, she seemed cautious. She felt that this illness was not serious enough to justify increased cortisone, which would risk retarding Nancy's growth. Of course, I knew the risk, but felt uneasy about withholding it. Dr. Wentworth had stated the need to double her daily dose of cortisone during illnesses, and I told Dr. Lynn that if she called Dr. Wentworth, I was sure she would increase Nancy's cortisone under these circumstances. I left for home in a very anxious state of mind. I knew in my heart that by morning Nancy would be back under emergency treatment. I intended to do just as the doctors told me to do, but still the fear would not leave.

Once home, Mark made the decision to send Jamie to stay at his mother's place for the night - just in case we had to leave suddenly with Nancy. I agreed. With Jamie cared for, there would be one less worry for me. My every thought right now was focused on Nancy's welfare.

My thoughts lingered for a moment on my Jamie. She was four years old - and such a good daughter! She could sense when my stress levels were building, and consistently showed a special sensitivity to my needs. She did most everything I asked of her without question. Jamie was more help to me in caring for Nancy than anyone would ever know. Whenever Nancy was in the middle of a seizure, or had to be rushed away for medical treatment, Jamie was careful to do exactly what I asked her to do. Whether the task at hand was to get herself together, or to get something for Nancy, I never once repeated myself nor was I left waiting. It became a routine, actually. In fact, Jamie moved a lot faster than any of the nurses I had observed over this period. It was as though I were the doctor giving the orders, and by my side was the best "nurse" around Jamie. I was proud that God gave her to me.

Since Nancy had already taken four ounces of glucose water at the clinic at five o' clock, I planned her next scheduled feeding for eight. I carefully lined up all her bottles for the night so they 'd be ready to go. At six o'clock I gave Nancy one ounce with medication, and at seven-thirty I repeated the procedure.

I decided I would feel better if I put Nancy down to sleep in her carriage - right next to my bed where I could hear her in case she awoke before my alarm went off. Mark wasn't too pleased with this arrangement. He couldn't see how any of us would get to sleep with her heavy breathing in our ears, not to mention the anxious burden of listening for her all night. But the carriage was roomy enough to serve as her bed, and after I elevated her head the breathing came much easier.

Because of the two ounces she'd already had between her regular feedings, it was nine o'clock before I fed Nancy again. Mark and I were encouraged to see her vigorously drinking down the required five ounces of liquid. My sense of foreboding was lifting. Surely now she would make it through the night!

Saturday, January 17, 1981

As soon as Nancy had settled down, we went to bed. At one o'clock I awoke and fed her five and-a-half ounces with medication. (I had let her go an extra hour because of medication and the previous feeding.) She drank well. I reset the alarm for four o'clock and went back to sleep.

At 2:00 a.m. however, Nancy woke me up. She was all stuffed up- extremely congested. I got out of bed and just held her, hoping to position her so she would clear up a little. But my anxiety had returned, and my hopes of keeping her home through the night were quickly fading. At that point Mark woke up. I told him she didn't sound good, but he assured me she would be all right and suggested I put her back to sleep. I did, but by 2:45 a.m. Nancy had begun to vomit. It seemed that everything she could possibly have inside her had come up, and still her stomach was rolling. For a moment I was relieved that she seemed to have rid herself of all the phlegm, and held hopes that she would now feel much better. But her breathing was shallow and she was no longer responding to me. Her pale color and lethargy told me that Nancy was in a bad way.

Mark then got up and carried Nancy to the kitchen, firmly telling me to calm down and stay quiet. For the first time it was nice to give him the responsibility. The moment finally came when he told me to call the Rescue and the ambulance. I called, then hurriedly readied myself to go with her.

The Rescue came quickly, within a few minutes. Although Mark was an EMT himself and had years of experience on calls, he left this case to the other men. "I've done a lot of CPR," he remarked, "but I don't want to do it on my own daughter." The Rescue squad then blew some oxygen across her face, and her color started to come back. She was coming around.

The ambulance arrived shortly after the Rescue. Once she was settled in the ambulance, Nancy continued to receive oxygen across her face and seemed more comfortable. At

4:00 a.m. Nancy was admitted to the UMASS Medical Intensive Care Unit.

    ** 1-17-81   Dis. 1-21-81
    Diagnosis:
    1. Congenital hypopit.
    2. Upper respiratory inf.
    3. Vomiting

The two residents on duty in the Trauma Room had treated Nancy before, so I didn't have as many questions to answer this time. I had brought all of all Nancy's medications with me in the fear that I would never remember all the ones she was on. When the nurse asked about Nancy's medications, I pulled out all the prescriptions and he copied them down. (This was the first time I had dealt with a male nurse, and I was impressed.)

Dr. Sizer and Dr. Louis were working on Nancy together. "When they told me she was dehydrated, I was shocked. I had been feeding her liquids every three to five hours - and now she was dehydrated? I quickly learned that it doesn't take long at all for an infant to dehydrate. Nancy was also quite lethargic and not responding very well. I had no doubt she was extremely ill and would have to be hospitalized.

The two residents were trying to locate a vein so they could start an I.V. on Nancy. This had always been a problem, but I allowed them to poke at her until my endurance crumbled. It was such an ordeal that I had to request that they send for the I.V. team. Dr. Louis seemed content just to keep trying various locations in Nancy's right arm, but Dr. Sizer was sticking needles in Nancy's feet as though she were a pincushion. The only place he didn't try was on her head she was too old for that. He would have kept on poking, too, if I hadn't firmly suggested that they call the I.V. team. Certainly Nancy would have to have an I.V., but I could no longer stand their jabbing and probing. Just because Nancy was not responding to pain didn't mean she wasn't hurting! Success in starting the I.V. on her had turned into a challenge to their competence, an ego trip. I was in no mood to play their games.

Soon a girl from the I.V. team arrived and examined Nancy's left arm, which had only been tried once. She found a vein, slipped the needle in, and bingo! It was up and running. I thanked her, hoping that perhaps the two residents had learned something that night.

Watching doctors sticking Nancy with needles in their attempt to find a vein was very difficult for me. I would tense up inside with every try, praying that this time it would work. I would relax after a vein was found, but there were still many times the vein would blow out after only a short time. Thankfully, most of the time the I.V. needle would manage to stay in for at least twenty-four hours. My general feeling was that I myself could do a better job. Certainly I was no professional, but after having watched so many I.V.s started I would have tried myself if I had been asked.

By 7:00 a.m., Nancy had been moved into the ICU. By around eight, Mark and I were able to return home for some rest. It was growing easier to leave Nancy. I knew the hospital procedures and I felt comfortable with the nurses, who loved her. I felt little worry about her being left in ICU.

Back at the house, the first thing I did was to call the clinic and speak with Dr. Lynn. I simply told her what had happened with Nancy, and requested that she be sure to let Dr. Matthew know. Even though I had disagreed with Dr. Lynn about increasing Nancy's cortisone, I did not make this call out of spite. Like all the other times I had called, this was simply to keep Dr. Matthew informed. At this point, I knew that if Nancy needed to be admitted it would be only to the University Hospital. Nancy's case was rare, and I felt the only one who could handle full responsibility while she needed hospital care was Dr. Wentworth. I was weary of the continual confusion that seemed to result when I merely tried to do what I was told with Nancy. First she would be treated at the clinic until her condition got bad enough to be admitted, then off we would go to UMASS Medical. Too many doctors were giving too many orders - it was a three-ring circus!

Monday, January 19, 1981
My mother had made plans to drive up to meet me this afternoon at UMASS Medical. She had decided it was time for her to come - not only for Nancy, but for me. Mothers! Always there when you need them. I was there for Nancy, and now my mother would be here for me. My mother came in around one o'clock and remarked how well Nancy looked. My mother, a nurse herself, could tell just by looking at her and at her surroundings that these nurses were giving Nancy excellent care. My mother had been in the profession for twenty years, teaching and practicing in state hospitals. She had risen to become a state inspector for nursing homes in Massachusetts. With her background, it was easy for her to tell that in this hospital Nancy and I were receiving good care.

After we had visited for a while, Dr. Wentworth came into the room. Since Nancy had been admitted on a Saturday morning, I hadn't seen her until this moment. I had no sooner introduced her to my mother than she fired her first question at me. "Why haven't you increased Nancy's cortisone?" I could hardly believe my ears. Her tone implied that I was a child who needed to be reprimanded for misunderstanding her instructions. I explained that I didn't know why, except that I had not been instructed to do so by any of the other doctors. Dr. Wentworth emphasized that when Nancy was ill like this, or not acting like herself, I was to go ahead with the cortisone increase without waiting for other instructions. In such cases Nancy needed it right away; it was what would make her better. At that point I would have loved to have a good scream and unload my feelings, but instead I agreed with Dr. Wentworth and held my peace. I had been through just about enough during the past two days. I knew I had tried my best to do everything I had been told, including increasing her cortisone. But the other doctors had put me off, saying her illness was not stressful enough to warrant it.

I did let Dr. Wentworth know that I wanted to bring Nancy to Children's Hospital in Boston for a second opinion. This was for my own sake. I deeply needed to feel better about all the effort I was putting in. Dr. Wentworth said she would give me the name of a doctor there whom she had been consulting with, but wanted me to wait until the growth hormone levels had been tested so we could provide more complete information. I agreed. I also wanted very much to give Nancy time to get well.

When Dr. Wentworth had gone, I couldn't keep the tears from my eyes. My mother comforted me, saying it would be all right. Dr. Wentworth had been tough on me, leaving me feeling like a student nurse who had given improper treatment to a patient. I was only Nancy's mother, trying to learn to take care of her as best I could. My mother assured me that Dr. Wentworth seemed like a very good doctor who knew what she was doing, but she also recognized that the way everything seemed to be going was hard on me. She encouraged me simply to do whatever Dr. Wentworth said, and in time everything would get better. I agreed, but right now I was overcome by the unfairness of having to accept the total blame for Nancy not getting proper treatment. I had suggested the cortisone increase; it was a doctor who had put off the idea.

Just then a nurse came to report that Nancy was being treated with antibiotics because of a bladder infection. They were about to move Nancy to the floor, the nurse said. She went on to say that tomorrow Nancy was scheduled for EEG testing and a CAT scan. Nancy had already had an EEG test done, but another had been ordered by Dr. Adams, who would see Nancy before she left. The CAT scan was to determine whether or not Nancy had a pituitary gland. I made it clear to the nurse that since the tests were scheduled so closely together, I did not want Nancy to be drugged more than once. (The EEG was set for 9:00 a.m. and the CAT scan for noon.) I requested that Nancy have natural sleep for the EEG, and understood that she would have to be drugged afterwards for the CAT scan. The nurse promised to relay my wishes to the doctor. I knew my request wasn't likely to be honored, but held onto the hope that someone would be intelligent enough to realize that administering anesthetics twice in such a short time frame was overdoing it. At least I had expressed my concern.

Tuesday, January 20, 1981
At 3:00 p.m. I entered UMASS Medical and approached the nurses' station. I found Nancy lying in her crib right next to the nurse's desk. One glance at her confirmed to me that they had put Nancy under for both tests without even consulting me. When her nurse spotted me, she came over to tell me that Nancy would be staying here until she woke up. I asked whether Nancy had been drugged for both tests, and she answered yes. She told me that Nancy had been taken down for the EEG test at 10:00 a.m. and the CAT scan for noon. I stated to her that there had been no reason to drug Nancy for both tests -that surely Nancy must have been still asleep when the EEG was done. Of course, the nurse was not free to comment, but she did agree with me.

One of the doctors came by and estimated that Nancy should be coming around by 5:00 or so. I replied that he'd be lucky if she was awake by midnight. It wasn't said entirely as a joke, either - but we did smile. Caring for Nancy was all I could handle right now; I had to put my anger behind me and use a little humor to keep myself from ending up in the state hospital next door. Humor would help preserve my sanity and defuse some of the anger for the time being.

I fed Nancy her bottle around five, but by 7:00 p.m. my patience had worn thin. She was still asleep. When the nurse came by, I told her I was about to leave and asked for the I.V. to be removed. I could see that it was infiltrating. She checked with the doctor about replacing the I.V. He answered that Nancy could come completely off it, so it came out. While she was there, the nurse asked me whether Nancy's eyes were normally crossed. I told her no - I was sure the drugs were affecting them. I drew strength from the thought that tomorrow I could take Nancy home. All I had to do was wait twenty-four hours to get her there.

I knew the hospital was a good one. I wouldn't be taking Nancy there if it weren't. I only wished they would listen to what I had to say. Every time I brought Nancy in, I felt all I was good for was to sign on the dotted line. Oh yes, I was allowed to talk -- but as to what they were hearing, there seemed to be a brick wall between us. I had no reservations concerning their competence as doctors; they had gone through all their schooling and were thoroughly updated in modem medicine. They were very knowledgeable people what I would call book-smart – but their course of action always followed the book. There seemed to be a lack of that good, intuitive common sense that comes with experience. I felt extremely uneasy whenever my intuition compelled me to question a resident's diagnosis or recommended procedure. When I did, I could feel a cold shoulder turned my way. I felt the snub, but knew I could not afford to let it silence me.

Wednesday, January 21, 1981
After lunch Mark, Jamie, and I headed to the hospital to bring Nancy home. When we arrived, the nurse told me that Nancy had been up since 6:00 a.m. and was growing fairly tired. Nancy had slept eighteen hours the day before, only waking up at midnight for her medication. It was no mystery to me why she had not napped.

Then Dr. Adams showed up with three residents to evaluate Nancy. He let me know that the EEG test had revealed no brain disorder, so they were assuming the seizures were hypoglycemic. This was no big relief to me; I already knew she was not suffering any damage from the seizures. My mother instincts told me she was okay, but I was content to let the record show she had been tested.

Dr. Adams proceeded to test Nancy's reflexes, hearing, and

eye contact. I let him know she had been up since 6:00 a.m. and was very tired, so he agreed to take that into consideration. He then picked up a small bell and rang it on both sides of Nancy's head. When she showed no quick response, he was not pleased. Dr. Adams advised me to have her hearing tested to make sure there was nothing wrong. I was not really concerned about it. But again, I would do as I was told.

Shortly after Dr. Adams left, Dr. Wentworth came in. Because we had missed Nancy's regular appointment at the clinic yesterday, the doctor wanted to perform a routine check on Nancy before we left. We reviewed Nancy's daily dosages of medication, and covered instructions about when to increase her cortisone. Dr. Wentworth again reminded me that Nancy would need to have testing done to measure how much growth hormone she was producing. It would require a hospital stay - and, of course, Nancy would have to be well in order to proceed.

Monday, January 26, 1981
During Nancy's follow-up appointment with Dr. Matthew, he commented that she looked good, but he noted that she still had some wheezing. He recommended starting her again on the ellixicon. I mentioned to him that her wheezing and coughing seemed to lessen when she was on increased dosages of hydrocortisone.

Dr. Matthew still had some concerns about me, and urged me to call him if I needed anything. It was true I was showing signs of stress, but I decided I would be all right. I assured him that if I needed his help I would ask him for it.

Tuesday, January 27, 1981
Nancy's 3:00 p.m. appointment with the Child Development Service concluded with the assessment that Nancy was developing well at ten months. They would check her again in another six months.

Wednesday, January 28, 1981

Dr. Wentworth called me in the morning with the news that she was going to try to get Nancy admitted today for the growth hormone testing. I was excited. I agreed that if we waited much longer, Nancy would likely get sick again. I told her that Nancy had been causing me some concern because she was eating poorly. Dr. Wentworth promised to call me back in the afternoon to let me know if our plans were confirmed.

I was developing an ability to sense when Nancy was headed toward another illness. No one else seemed to understand this sixth sense. But sure enough, there was a pattern to it. Three days before Nancy would come down with something, I would experience a "knowing" that I would soon be at the doctor's with her again. I had no solid proof, of course, but each time I had to take her in with an illness I could count back three days to the time I started sensing she was about to get sick.

Nancy was eating fairly well today, but not nearly as well as I would have liked. Her wheezing made eating difficult for her. I fought back fear that it would be another illness instead of the hormone testing that she was about to be admitted for.

Around mid-afternoon Dr. Wentworth called to say that they were unable to secure a bed for Nancy. Naturally I was disappointed, but Dr. Wentworth promised to try again for tomorrow. I did confess to her that Nancy was not feeling her best. She reminded me to double her cortisone if she stopped eating or became ill. I readily assured her that I would not forget.

At 5:00 p.m. I got ready to feed Nancy. Her meal was two tablespoons of a vegetable and two tablespoons each of meat and dessert. I sat down to begin feeding her, but as time passed it became evident that Nancy was accepting nothing. I changed the variety of food; she still refused to eat. Nancy didn't even want her bottle. After an hour-and-a-half of these attempts, I finally gave up. It was now 7 :00 p.m. and I was exhausted from just trying to get her to take one bite. I increased her cortisone and called Dr. Wentworth at her home to let her know what was going on.

I was weeping over the phone as I asked her how one was supposed to feed a child who needs nourishment and refuses to eat. Dr. Wentworth told me to bring her down to UMASS Medical. She would call ahead to inform them we were coming My sister-in-law drove us to the hospital, with the understanding that Mark would come to pick me up after he got out of work. By now we had developed a routine with our friends and family.

No one ever knew when Nancy and I might need to go to the hospital, but someone was always ready to take us with no questions asked. I could only focus on Nancy - Jamie came next, the house and my husband. He was not handling it very well and I was functioning. I just didn't know when or if things would ever become "normal." He seemed disappointed with this "crisis" lifestyle at times, which left me feeling inadequate as a wife. But when it came to caring for Nancy, I had to put everyone's needs including my own - on the back burner until the family was back to normal.

> "U. Mass. 1-21-81
> Chief complaint:
> Dish. Diagnosis:
> Dich. 2-3-81
> NOT EATING
> 1. Addisonian crisis
> 2. Panhypopit.
> 3. Upper respirator infection"
> To be released on 2-2-81
> Phycosocial

In the emergency room we met up with Dr. Louis and Dr. Sizer. As they proceeded to take a poke at Nancy's veins, I explained to them what was going on. (The hours I spent telling Nancy it would be okay are too numerous to tell.)

Finally they found a vein in her head, just above her right eye. She was actually getting too old to put an I.V. in her head, but they planned to keep a good watch on it during the night.

By 11 :00 p.m. Nancy had been transferred upstairs to the pediatric floor. She was settled in, but before I left I wanted a good look at her I.V. It didn't look too good. I alerted the nurse, who went to have Dr. Louis come in and look at it. Dr. Louis thought it looked all right, and assured me she planned to keep a close watch on it through the night. After the doctor was gone, I confided to the nurse my fear that surely the vein could not last. I had seen I.V.s enough times on Nancy to know when the needle should be pulled. The nurse agreed that most likely I was right. She could see that the vein didn't look very good, but it was too early for the doctor to say. She promised to keep an eye on it, though. I knew that by now Nancy had earned a reputation for her hard-to-reach veins. The last thing they were going to do was to pull it early. I shook my head and went home.

Thursday, January 29, 1981
It was Mark's day off, so we were planning a leisurely afternoon. Mark spent many of his days off now visiting Nancy. Before we went to the hospital today I called Dr. Matthew to let him know Nancy had been admitted and was supposed to be tested for human growth hormone on Friday. When we arrived on the pediatric floor, Dr. Louis was standing at the nurses' station. We breezed by her with a quick hello and went straight to Nancy's room. Nancy was awake. She turned over as I approached, revealing the biggest swollen right eye I'd ever seen! Mark wanted to know what happened. I quickly explained that the I.V. had infiltrated, adding that I was certainly going to ask Dr. Louis about it.

Mark stayed with Nancy while I searched down the hall; but Dr. Louis was nowhere to be found. As soon as I came back to the room, a nurse entered behind me, explaining that the I.V. had infiltrated. She told me Nancy's eye had been fine this morning when she awoke, but after she had napped again, she had awakened with it swollen. The nurse said she had tried to keep Nancy from sleeping on that side, saying that it doesn't take long for the swelling to set in. She told us that tests had been ordered just so they could rule out infection. I knew as well as she did that there was no infection, but accepted her explanation. I told her I had gone to search for Dr. Louis to just ask if it was the I.V. and she was gone. The nurse said Dr. Louis was reprimanded because she did not keep a close watch on it and the head doctor was quite upset that this happened.

Nancy was a sight - her right eye was so swollen she could not see out of it. As many times as I tried to get my feelings across to the doctors, I was not listened to. Instead, I had to wait and listen to their excuses why it happened. I would bite my tongue and never said "If you'd only listen to me" or "I told you so." It really wasn't worth my time; it was a lesson and I prayed that some day they would listen to me.

Friday, January 30, 1981
Dr. Matthew had agreed to meet us at UMASS around 4:00 p.m. to check on Nancy and me. I was encouraged about the growth hormone testing which was about to be performed on Nancy. Finally, we would have some missing information on her condition. Perhaps it would bring a quick ending to this whole nightmare.

At around 2:00 p.m. I went to the hospital. The nurse put Nancy in my arms to hold. As I sat in the rocking chair, I carefully watched the place in Nancy's arm where the I.V. line was running in. There was so much blood that had to be drawn from Nancy that they couldn't perform it with a regular I.V. setup. She had to have a main line so the vein would not blow. Over the next eight hours they would repeatedly draw blood - all at the specific times listed on the chart attached to her crib.

As I held Nancy, I felt the hopefulness that comes when one more step of progress is being made. Although I couldn't understand fully what they were doing for her, I felt confident that eventually she would get better. I was aware of a load of guilt inside me, a nagging sense that perhaps the hospital was the best place for Nancy. Feelings of failure and inadequacy were building up pressure inside me, slowly eroding my confidence in my own ability to care for Nancy properly. Every time I would get sure of myself, something would happen and I would feel like a failure. Over and over, just as I'd begin to get comfortable with Nancy at home, she would get sick. I felt as though I just couldn't do anything right. Since Nancy had to be fed every five hours, a full night's sleep was very rare for me except when she was hospitalized. I was becoming physically and mentally exhausted.

I was happy to see Dr. Matthew when he came in. Perhaps he was a doctor, but I found him comfortingly down-to-earth, like the nurses. He would explain Nancy's treatments and conditions to me at my own level. At UMASS - in contrast - every time I listened to a doctor I'd have to go ask a nurse what it was the doctor was trying to tell me. I knew that I was by no means lacking intelligence. When I was with some of the doctors, however, I definitely found myself questioning theirs!

After Dr. Matthew had looked over Nancy's charts, he came in to see her and to review the procedures being used on her. I had already put Nancy back in her crib earlier so she could sleep. I felt the less I disturbed her, the better.

Dr. Matthew and I stepped outside Nancy's room to chat so we would not wake her. Even
though I was comfortable about the care Nancy was receiving in the hospital, I knew it wasn't pleasant for her. And that pained me even more.

Dr. Matthew remarked that the chart written up by the doctor was very good- even impressive. The chart had evidently been written up by a Dr. Moore, a female resident whom I had not met. I knew Nancy was not a simple case, but I was content to leave the technical work to the experts.

Since Dr. Matthew was ready to leave, and I knew that Tom would be waiting outside to drive me home, we walked out together. It was a nice change to have a social conversation for once. Dr. Matthew mentioned that he was considering opening a practice in the Gardner area. My eyes lit up as I told him how nice that would be. I assured him he already had his first patient. It was a relief to know that at least he was considering moving to this area. When we parted, I told him I'd be in to see him on Monday. I needed to talk.

Once again I climbed into the car with Tom. This was just one of many rides home he had provided for me. He was always so good about picking me up at the hospital so I'd be sure of having a way to get home. I felt very grateful for the friendship of Tom and Lisa. They were true friends.

FEBRUARY 1981

Sunday, February I, 1981
Now I knew I was running around too much. My whole life consisted of doctors, hospital, and home. I had come down with a cold and I could feel myself burning out.

In the afternoon I went in to see Nancy. She had come out of ICU and was back in the same room with Johnny. There was another child next to her who suffered from bronchitis, and one directly across from her who was the saddest case I had ever seen. The boy was fourteen years old, he measured perhaps all of two-and-a-half feet tall, and his head was larger than a watermelon. His body was very thin and frail, with no hair at all. All he could do was moan. I will never forget him.

Everything was starting to pile up on me now. I was battling a cold, I had nearly no time at home, and to top it off, Nancy didn't appear to be getting any better. It seemed all I was doing was taking and giving out information to doctors, nurses, family, and friends. And to have to watch these other children suffer as well - whether it was more or less than my daughter – was really depressing me. I needed a break.

Nancy was doing fairly well so far except for the problems she had with eating. Certainly I was aware of how much Nancy had been through, but that nagging sense that she was on the way to being sick again just drained me. I didn't stay with her very long this time; I was plain tired out. I needed to go home.

As I was leaving, the head pediatric doctor stopped me to give a report on how Nancy was doing. He felt she could go home tonight if I wanted to take her. Without warning, I found myself beginning to cry. The shock of overwhelming pressure overflowed inside me and I just couldn't contain it anymore. I explained to him that I had set a doctor's appointment for myself tomorrow because of all I'd been through with Nancy. I explained that I felt too emotionally unstable to take her home this soon. I told him I was going to talk things through with Dr. Matthew and try to get some issues straightened out in my mind. (I had discovered that this stress on the immediate family was the reason the word "Phycosocial" had been added to Nancy's admission report.) He understood and agreed. It was all right, he said.

I had no intention of taking Nancy home just now. If I were put on the spot I knew I would have had to give a direct refusal. My bad feelings were not toward Nancy, but had to do with a sense of inadequacy to care for her properly. I needed to hear someone I respected tell me I was not doing anything wrong - to be convinced that what was happening to me was normal. I longed for assurance that I wasn't doing any harm to Nancy. For the past five months my life had revolved totally around her, and now depression had definitely overtaken me.

Monday, February 2, 1981

It was extremely unusual for me to be going to a clinic appointment just for myself. But at 9:45 a.m. that's exactly what I did. As Dr. Matthew and I talked through my issues about Nancy's care, I let him know that my strongest inclination right now was to go over to the state hospital located next door to UMASS and just check myself in. (Actually, it was that kind of humorous, tongue-in-cheek statement which was helping to keep me away from there.) The doctor recognized that Nancy's condition was very difficult for me - as her mother- to handle. He reassured me that my feelings were normal under the circumstances, impressing on me that I was a very good mother.

To be told I was doing a good job was just the medicine I needed to combat the guilt that had been weighing on me. Dr. Matthew went on to say that so far, all of Nancy's admissions had been absolutely necessary. She needed to be in the hospital. He agreed that, ideally, home is the best place for any child, but said that for now we had to accept the unusual circumstances of Nancy's case. His encouragement was all I needed; I could feel the weight of guilt lifting.

Later in the day I decided I was ready to bring Nancy home. But when I arrived at the hospital, I saw that she didn't look all that great. The nurse told me that Nancy had been vomiting, and that she would have to stay another night. She explained that Nancy had not been eating well, surmising that most likely the stress of her recent testing had thrown her system off. I hadn't expected to be going home without Nancy. But I would summon my patience and come back to get her tomorrow after supper. Surely another 24 hours would tell us whether there was still anything ·wrong.

Tuesday, February 3, 1981
I returned to UMASS at around three o'clock so I could be there for Nancy's supper. I wanted to see for myself how she was eating. The nurse described for me what a hard time she had feeding Nancy, and how Dr. Moore had finally taken over and had managed to get Nancy to finish her bottle.

It felt good to know that a doctor had personally taken the time to feed Nancy, but I also sensed that the difficulty with her feeding would be best handled at home. I knew something was wrong; there always was when Nancy refused food or had difficulty eating. I would take her home where she belonged and would find a way to deal with her feedings there.

Wednesday, February 4, 1981

In the morning, Nancy refused to eat a single bite of anything. I did manage to get her medications down, but that was all. I called the clinic and arranged an appointment with Dr. Matthew for 10:20 a.m. Nancy had not yet reached the stage of having a seizure, but I knew that with no food inside her it would not be long. I tried to get some glucose with Pedialyte into her, and had contented myself with her little sips. She vomited just before we left for the doctor's office.

At the clinic, Dr. Matthew checked Nancy over and then left the office for a few minutes. I could judge by his actions that Nancy was sick. By now I could nearly tell what the doctor was thinking just by observing him. When Dr. Matthew returned, he informed me that Nancy was suffering from "viral gastrotonitis," and would have to be admitted. Tears came to my eyes. I told him she had just left UMASS yesterday. Now would she have to go back? He answered no. At this I gave him a puzzled look, and he told me that Nancy could go to Holden District Hospital, where he could treat her for this himself. I was relieved and comforted. Holden was closer to home, and she would be directly under Dr. Matthew's care.

Nancy's blood sugar was checked just before we left, and I was instructed to bring her to Holden District Hospital for a three o'clock admission. I still had a little time to go home and put some things together before going in with Nancy. Although going to Holden meant I'd have to stay longer with her because she would be new to the nurses there, I was not overly concerned.

> Holden District Hospital
> 2-4-81 "Panhypo. 2. Viral gastroenteritis asthma"
> 2-11-81 Discharged

When we arrived at three o'clock, I stopped first at the emergency room, which was my custom at UMASS. There they told me that we could go right up to Pediatrics, where the nurses were waiting for us. What a turn-around! I was used to waiting in the E.R. for hours, and here we were, being treated like people rather than numbers!

A nurse led us up to Pediatrics, where they gave Nancy a crib and started the admission procedure. Everyone came to us. The admissions personnel came up to the floor to .get the information they needed. The entire process went very smoothly - I was impressed.

Nancy had been vomiting off and on, but now she seemed all right. Soon Dr. Matthew arrived and started the I.V. on Nancy. I sat down to fill out forms and answer all the questions the nurse had for me. Compared to UMASS, this place was heaven. The ward was small (14 beds), and the nurses ' station was located directly across from Nancy. All beds were visible to the nurses' station, whereas at UMASS the children were tucked away in separate rooms, the way it would be on an adult floor. Between my attention and Dr. Matthew's care, I felt that this place would work out just fine for Nancy.

The nurses were concerned about Nancy's seizures, so I had to explain to them what typically would happen to her, and what I had learned to do for it. Seizures frighten people, just as Nancy's had frightened me. But when you've come through it and treated it as many times as I had with Nancy, the fear leaves you. The anxiety is always there, but the emotions I had attached to it all were beginning to stabilize. I had noticed how she always· came back to normal as soon as her blood sugar level came up.

Nancy stayed in Holden Hospital for a week, mostly because of the vomiting. Each time she would seem to be doing better, she would later have a setback. After quite a bit of observation, I was able to suggest to the nurses that Nancy's vomiting was caused by the liquid medication. Every time she was given the Elixicon for the wheezing, she would vomit. Eventually, we got her off the Elixicon, and by Wednesday the 11th, she was all ready to go home.

During Nancy's stay I met a lot of new people - mostly the nurses. Nancy was a beautiful baby with a sweet personality, and soon found herself the darling of the hospital. In addition, her medical disability was so rare that she attracted many curious nurses who just wanted to check her out. I will never forget the nurse who came in one afternoon to ask me, "When will the transplant be done?" I couldn't help laughing! I wasn't trying to be rude, but it was clear that whatever rumors were going around had to be pretty amazing! I explained that there wouldn't be any transplant, but did tell this nurse that I was waiting to hear about the possibility of Nancy receiving injections of human growth hormone in the near future. I also told her that we didn't know yet whether or not Nancy had a pituitary gland.

Friday, February 13, 1981
At 11:00 a.m. I was scheduled to see Dr. Matthew in order to learn how to tube-feed Nancy.
This was strictly in preparation for an emergency situation, but still it was a good thing for me to learn. I had no intention whatsoever of actually doing this on Nancy at home, but if it were needed as a last resort, at least I would have the knowledge.

A visiting nurse was also at the clinic today, and Dr. Matthew urged me to have her come to my home to help with Nancy. The idea of sharing the daily responsibility for Nancy was difficult for me to accept. I had been with Nancy constantly from the beginning. Nothing went into her mouth that I did not put there. It was true I had become somewhat obsessed with her care, which was a great source of stress, but who could possibly take proper care of her at home besides me?
Finally, however, I gave in. The visiting nurse would come to our house on the 19th to check on us and see how we were.

Over the weekend, Nancy fared pretty well. She did vomit once, but I knew it was a reaction to the Elixicon she was being given to treat her wheezing, so I lived with it. Nancy's bowel movements were becoming hard, however, so I called and spoke with Dr. Stem. He told me to give her some prosobie and a suppository- and, of course, to call him if I felt the need.

Nancy seemed stable, but as time progressed she grew congested, with a definite increase in her coughing. I didn't enjoy the noise, but considered it a good sign that at least she was moving the phlegm.

Wednesday, February 18, 1981
Nancy was not eating. She was drinking her bottle easily, but she would have nothing to do with solid food. I took her temperature - it was 100.4 degrees. Again I called the clinic. Dr. Thomas arranged to see Nancy at 11 a.m. By now I was growing disgusted with this pattern. The simple joy of having Nancy at home for a solid day seemed nearly out of reach.

We saw Dr. Thomas, as planned, at eleven. "Sick, temp. 100.4 - up cortisol. 2.5 pm - 5 mg. am – no signs of infection." He told me to call if I needed help.

Thursday, February 19, 1981
Nancy's bowel movements had turned black. I had spoken on the phone with Dr. Matthew about this the night before, and he requested that I save Nancy's stool sample to bring in with her at 10:00 a.m. the next day. There was hardly a single body function of Nancy's that I wasn't monitoring now. I was growing tired.

When Dr. Matthew checked the stool sample today, he agreed that it was black. His testing showed no evidence of blood in the stool, however, so I could relax a little. "Black stool - was a Negative. Eating and doing well otherwise."

Dr. Matthew took the time to talk with me for a while. It was plain to him that I was burning out. I told him that Mark and I were planning to go out tonight, so I would be all right.

The visiting nurse dropped by in the afternoon. I told her that Nancy's increased congestion was troubling me. She listened to her breathing and concluded that Nancy was indeed congested, but because it was moving she should be all right. I was able to talk through a number of things with her, and was greatly encouraged just by the fact that she listened. I shared with her my foreboding that Nancy was on the way to getting ill again, and that another hospital stay loomed on the horizon. But I was comfortable with Nancy for now, so there was nothing to do but wait.

This was the night that Mark and I had made plans to go grocery shopping together in Worcester. At six o'clock, when Mark's mother planned to come over to babysit, we would be on our way. Grocery shopping may not sound like an exciting event, but I hadn't done it for over a month. We had gotten through the month because Mark's mother was doing most of it, and we were just picking up our immediate needs at a convenience store. It would be a treat just to be able to stock my own cupboards! We were definitely not running a "normal" household!

It was around four o'clock when I began to sense inwardly that the shopping trip was not going to happen. It hit me just as I had started to think about feeding the girls their supper and getting myself ready to leave. I tried to deny what I was feeling, reasoning within myself that Nancy had seen Dr. Matthew only this morning and the nurse had checked her this afternoon. Surely, I told myself, Nancy would be fine without me for a few hours. And I really needed - really wanted -to get out of the house with Mark for a change. I was determined to ignore my sixth sense and just go. I told Mark we would be leaving around six, right after Nancy had been fed.

It was around 4:15 p.m. that Nancy began to cough. This wasn't just an occasional bark; it was non-stop. "What's going on?" I huffed to myself. All these months there had been a cool-mist vaporizer running in her room. I was doing everything humanly possible to follow doctors' instructions, and now she was coughing uncontrollably. When it had continued for a solid 30 minutes, I called the clinic. Dr. Lynn got on the line and I described what was going on. She assured me Nancy would be all right, just to watch her' and call if there was any change. "But I was supposed to go out grocery shopping tonight," I told her, "and now I can't even do that!" I could not keep the anger out of my voice, and Dr. Lynn knew it. We finally hung up with the agreement that if there was any change, I would call her again.

Nancy stopped coughing around 5:00 p.m. I was pulled in twenty different directions and couldn't stop running around like a nut. Mark kept trying to reassure me that Nancy would be all right. I wanted to believe that, so I did my best to feed her so we could leave by six. Nancy refused to eat, but drank her bottle. I figured she was on enough liquids to be all right for now. I would go ahead and go shopping.

All that was left to do was wait for my mother-in-law to arrive. In the meantime, I decided to check Nancy's temperature. She was on a schedule of Tylenol doses to keep a slight 100.4° temperature in check, and just before we took off I wanted to take a reading and give her the next dose of Tylenol. I was mad to see the thermometer-reading shoot up to 102° within just a few seconds. And that was while she still had Tylenol in her. I told Mark to forget going; there was no way I could leave now.

I called Dr. Lynn again to report that Nancy's temperature was now up to 102. What could be wrong? She simply told me to give her Tylenol and call again if Nancy continued to get worse. My emotions were spinning out of control now. I replied that Nancy was already on Tylenol, and she obviously wasn't getting any better- she had been running a temp for two days! I lamented that just when I finally had a chance to get out for a change, now I couldn't even do that. Dr. Lynn simply said, "We can't be a babysitter for you." I told her that I didn't need a babysitter! I admitted to her that I was upset, and apologized - for what I had no idea - but I did apologize. We hung up. I often found myself apologizing to anyone I talked to - always saying that I was sorry.

When Mark's mother arrived, we had to explain to her what was going on. She urged us to go anyway, protesting that she would be all right under the circumstances. But Mark knew I was not about to go. My thoughts were on no one else but Nancy. At the moment she looked all right, but with Nancy there could always be a sudden turn-around.

The phone rang. It was Dr. Matthew, wanting to know what was going on. Naturally, I began to cry, and he responded ·with assurances that Nancy would be fine, and that he would see her in the morning. But I was still fuming, and unloaded my frustration about having to ditch my plans to get a change of scenery and go out. He, too, urged me to go. I also told him that I was upset about Dr. Lynn's comment that they were not my babysitter. Nancy would be fine, he repeated. I said no. Dr. Matthew told me to just keep the humidifier running, and to leave her in Pampers only if her temperature stayed high. Again, he assured me Nancy would be fine, and he would see her at 10:00 a.m. tomorrow. He wanted to know if I would be all right, and I replied yes.

Nancy seemed stable, but nevertheless I was keeping a constant watch on her. Throughout the night her temperature fluctuated between 102 and 104. I spent the whole time in Nancy's room. What sleep I got was on the hardwood floor.

Mark wasn't happy with the way I was handling this. I understood his disgust, but on the other hand, he wasn't offering to help me out, either. And even if he had, I would have told him to just forget it. Given the state I was in, anyone else with intentions to take care of Nancy would have had to firmly take over and command me to get some sleep, or absolutely insist that I go out and get a break. No one ever pushed that far, so I was allowed to control each situation. I also thought it was a burden for Mark, so the less he did the less guilty I would feel.

Friday, February 20, 1981
I brought Nancy in to see Dr. Matthew at 10:00 a.m. as planned. She was still running a temperature, and I related to the doctor everything that had taken place last evening after we had talked by phone. When he had listened carefully to Nancy's chest, he told me he needed a chest X-ray on her, and asked me to bring her out to the lab.

Whenever Nancy was being tested for infections or having blood work done, I had a practice of holding my peace and quietly waiting for the results. I rarely felt the need to ask questions; Dr. Matthew and I understood one another well enough so that our conversations were brief. It was a good relationship—one of trust. I didn't have to justify my actions to him, and I didn't expect him to explain his to me. It was a cooperation governed by honesty and openness.

When we got to the lab, Dr. Matthew began writing out the order for a chest X-ray. I would need to stay with Nancy during the X-ray to help out. It was necessary to seat her in an uncomfortable position, and she bawled through the whole ordeal. Then they had to place a chest form around her. It's a device made of plastic, designed to hold a squirming child in place just long enough for an X-ray. Nancy wasn't all that still, but it was good enough.

After the X-rays were taken, I knew it was going to take awhile to develop them. Dr. Matthew had other patients to see while we were waiting, so we settled down as comfortably as we could in the waiting area next to the lab. Dr. Matthew wanted me to bring Nancy in the following day at 10 a.m. for an informal check - nothing that needed to be entered with the receptionist.

Dr. Stern came over to us as we sat in the waiting area and

asked, "How does Nancy seem to you?" "Fine, now," I replied. "A lot better than she was last night." Dr. Stern said, "Okay," and left.

When Dr. Matthew had the X-ray results, he sat me down in his office. "Nancy does have double pneumonia," he said. "There is a little on each lung. It's not bad, so she can stay home." Tears stung my eyes again - now I was frightened. He described how I was to make a tent over her crib and put the cool mist under it, because she would need a lot of moisture.

"Okay," I responded, "I'll do it, but just how bad is she going to get? Will she be okay?"
He said, "Yes, she'll be okay."
"Is it going to get worse?" I wanted to know.
"Yes," he responded, "it's got to get worse before it gets better." I told him I wasn't going to make it. He told me I would. I promised to try.

I asked him, "If Nancy has to be admitted, does it have to be at UMASS?" He told me no, that she could go to Holden, although Holden was packed right now. Even so, if Nancy did have to be hospitalized, they did have a bed for her, he said. "But what if they fill that bed?" I asked. He told me that Nancy's name was on it, but they would only admit her if she really needed it. Nancy would be fine at home; the bed was there only if she really needed it.

After a short period of silence, I protested, "It's not going to work!"
"It will," he said.
"It won't!"
"It will," he repeated. Dr. Matthew then gave me a prescription for Amoxicillin - a liquid -along with instructions about when to give it. As he turned to leave the room, he smiled. "Don't sabotage us," he said. "I won't," I promised meekly. I knew what he meant. Just because there was a bed didn't automatically mean Nancy could have it.

Doctor's notes: "2-20 - pneumonia - admit if needed."

On the ride home, I spoke firmly to Nancy. "Dr. Matthew said you're going to make it, so you're going to," I told her. As we rode, my mind flooded with recent and frightening memories of past emergency admissions. By the time we reached home, I was in tears.

The house was empty when we arrived, and I felt as though the world was caving in around me. I busied myself getting Nancy's room prepared. I made a little tent and placed her in the crib. I even set up a portable T.V. on her dresser to keep her occupied. I left the room, once again in tears, and called Dr. Matthew. I wept aloud, protesting to him that I couldn't do it. I was banging my foot against the wall as I talked. I predicted glumly that she would vomit as soon as I gave her the liquid medicine. He was sure she wouldn't, but in the event she did, I could call. "She'll be okay; she will," he stated. "Remember we're here if she needs us."

After awhile, I calmed down a little. Dr. Matthew knew how frightened I was, and took the time to reassure me that they would be there. He reminded me once again that if she needed the hospital, she could go.

When Mark came home with Jamie, I broke the news that Nancy had pneumonia. I told him I had to go out to the pharmacy to pick up her medication. Since Mark's mother was planning to come over, I asked him if he would give her some money to buy us groceries. There was no way I could go shopping now.

Just as I was leaving, Mark's mother pulled in. I simply waved and told her that Nancy was in the house. I couldn't talk; it was all I could do to keep from crying again.

When I arrived home from the pharmacy, Mark told me that his mother had taken Jamie with her to go get us some groceries. He commented that Nancy seemed to be doing fine. I looked in on her and she did look great. When I gave her the Amoxicillin, she took it well with no vomiting. Up to this point, Nancy seemed to be doing well on fluids. I began to feel a little more secure about her.

It was just before dark when I began to feel nervous again. I was haunted by the fear that she might start dehydrating and turn blue, as she had done before. I told Mark that keeping Nancy here at home just wasn't going to work. Mark replied, "She's doing all right. Don't worry; she'll be fine." I had heard those words several times already today, and somehow they did nothing for me. I tried to explain to him my view of the situation. Perhaps Nancy had tolerated the first dose of Amoxicillin, I argued, but she was going to vomit the next one - I just knew it. There was nothing anyone could say to convince me otherwise. I warned Mark to just wait and see. In the meantime, my mother-in-law· and Jamie arrived home from their shopping trip loaded with groceries. I couldn't thank her enough. She also offered to take Jamie home with her for the night in case we had to run to the hospital with Nancy. We agreed, and I got my little sweetheart ready to go spend the night with her grandmother.

Mark and I ate supper together, just enjoying some time to relax after a long day. At about six o'clock I mentioned to Mark once again how certain I was that Nancy would vomit up her seven o'clock dose of Amoxicillin. I told him I was going to call the doctor. He said, "You're crazy at least wait until she does vomit." I complained to him that no one believed me, and that maybe I could bring Nancy to the doctor for her next dose, so he could see for himself that I wasn't making her vomit. I was filled with insecurities about telling them how sick Nancy's medicine kept making her.

It seemed as though no one believed me. I was sure that everyone secretly thought I was just making it up. Well, this time I wanted a doctor to see it with his own eyes. Mark grumbled that it was a stupid idea. But, he added, I was just going to do what I set my mind on anyway, so why ask him?

Around 6:30 I called the doctor's office and got Dr. Thomas. I told him Nancy was going to vomit when I gave her the Amoxicillin, and asked him what I should do.
"Did she vomit?" he questioned me.
I replied, "No, but she's going to."
He advised, "Let's just take one thing at a time."
I told him, "If I bring Nancy in and let you watch her take the medicine, you can see for yourself."

I could tell he thought I was crazy; there was no question about that. Dr. Thomas insisted that I wait until seven, give Nancy the Amoxicillin, and if she did vomit I could call him.
"Okay," I said, "I'll talk to you at seven."
"Only if she vomits," he reminded me.
"All right," I countered, " but she 's going to."

I knew Mark thought I was wacked out, but I let him know that this time, Nancy was NOT going to be rushed out in the middle of the night. I couldn't imagine Nancy making it through the night at home. But still, who can predict the future?

I waited until seven, got Nancy's medicine, and methodically picked her up out of her crib. I carefully sat her down with me in the rocking chair, and called for Mark to come to her room and watch us. I wanted him to verify that I did nothing to make Nancy vomit. There was a special spoon that had been provided to measure properly and keep the liquid from spilling when it was administered. I carefully filled this spoon and put it to Nancy's mouth. She had barely got a taste of it on her lips when she vomited all over the place. Case dismissed! Now maybe someone would listen to me.

I waited awhile, thinking Nancy might drink from her bottle, but she refused. I set her back in the crib and went to call Dr. Thomas back. I reported that Nancy had, indeed, vomited. I told him that she hadn't gotten any medication into her and that she refused to eat. He replied, "Okay, bring her in."

As we got ready to go, it was plain that Mark was not at all pleased. I admitted that the house had become a three-ring circus, but I could only do so much as a wife and mother. All I knew was that Nancy should have been sent to the hospital in the first place. I shouldn't have had to prove to everyone that she couldn't be treated at home. We arrived at the hospital around eight o'clock.

> Holden District Hospital
> 2-20-81 "Panhypopit. 2. Bilateral pneumonia."
> Disch. 2-22-81 U. Mass. Med. ICU

We brought Nancy straight up to Pediatrics, where the nurses took over and began to get her settled in. The place was full; there were more tents than I had ever seen. Though the nurses were extremely busy, somehow I knew Nancy was in good hands.

Dr. Thomas came in, checked Nancy over, and told us he was going to attempt to start an I.V. on her. He said he would only make two tries. If those failed, he would call in someone else. He made his two tries and was unable to find a vein. Shortly after that, Dr. Stem came in and put the I.V. needle straight in. It was an excellent job; I was impressed. Dr. Stem explained that they would be giving her antibiotics as well as glucose (sugar water) through the I.V. The nurse asked the doctors if they wanted Nancy under a tent, but they said no. I commented to them that Dr. Matthew had told me to give her a lot of moisture at home, but they didn't respond to this. I was extremely tired and didn't have the energy to question them further.

As we were all standing around waiting for the nurses to settle Nancy in, Mark made the comment to the doctors, "She looks fine to me!" The nurses looked up at me, and then to Mark. The doctors just shrugged their shoulders. I didn't quite believe Mark had made the comment, but I was determined to let their feelings slide past me. I knew Nancy needed hospital care and I was going to see she got it.

After Nancy was comfortable, we left for home. Mark was still upset with me, saying, "I don't know why you had to do that!" I replied that I would just go back in the morning to see how she was doing. I told him I knew she needed to be there, and this time, I wasn't fooling around. I let him know I was determined that Nancy was going to be taken care of on time, instead of waiting until the last minute to be rushed in as critical.

Saturday, February 21, 1981
I arrived at the hospital early the next morning, around 7:30. I found that Nancy had been moved and was now under a tent. One of the nurses came over and explained that she had Nancy put under a tent because she didn't sound good at all. She also told me that she had been trying to feed her with no success. I said I would try to get her to drink something. Rather than move Nancy from the moisture of the tent, I got under it with a bottle so I could feed her. She certainly didn't look well, and still would not drink. I tried talking to her, but there was no response. All she could do was sleep.

By eight o'clock, Dr. Matthew arrived. He greeted me with a cheery good morning. I told him I was sorry for my outburst. He told me not to worry. When he checked Nancy over, he started looking a little nervous. Dr. Willis came over then and took a turn listening to Nancy's chest. I could tell it was bad without either of them saying a word. Dr. Matthew told me they would have to get some blood from her to test her blood gas level. I would have to wait, which was nothing new to me; I did it often enough at UMASS. Since the nurses were extremely busy and space was tight, it was only natural for me to step in and help. Dr. Matthew began the procedure for drawing blood, but it seemed like forever (probably a good fifteen minutes) before he hit a vein. We were both upset and frustrated, because we knew the vein was actually there. But all her veins tended to roll too much, making the job extremely difficult. Patience was strong - it had to be.

Despite all the poking being done, Nancy did not budge. There was no sign of discomfort; she just laid there. We both knew it was not a good sign. I was always comforted by Nancy's crying and fussing when she was getting poked with needles, because it was a sign of wellness. Her lack of response scared me, and I could tell it unnerved Dr. Matthew, too. "She's bad," I commented to him. "Yes," he replied, "but I have to get the blood to see what's going on." I offered up a silent prayer, and finally the blood was drawn.

The blood was rushed to the lab for testing, and all we could do was to wait for the results. We talked. a little, but I could see that Dr. Matthew was anxious for the analysis to come back. It seemed like only a short time before he was handed the results. A smile spread across his face. All indications were good, and we could be happy. He told me he was going to write up more orders for Nancy, assuring me that he would be nearby all weekend since he was on call. He urged me to try my best to get some more fluids down her. From here on, he remarked, we would just have to see what happened.

As soon as Dr. Matthew had finished writing up the orders, the nurses came right over and started the changes. The head nurse said, "Forget this. We've got to get Nancy moved so we can work." So we moved Nancy and just about everything else. It was hectic. The nurse thanked me for what I was able to do for them, but by now it was second nature to me. I had learned a lot since Nancy was born.

The day passed quickly, and I watched the first shift nurses welcome the end of their workday. When Mark came by at the end of his shift, I briefed him on Nancy's condition, proposing that I wanted to stay the night. He was not in favor of it. I argued that she had only been awake twice that day, for a minute each time. I wanted her to know I was here with her. He gave in, but only reluctantly. He still felt I should be at home. I assured him I would be all right. I tried to explain why I felt I had to stay - not so much for myself as for Nancy. Of all Nancy's hospital admissions, this was the one I felt most strongly about. I had to stay; she needed me now more than ever.

I asked Mark if he would drop off a change of clothes for me in the morning on his way to work, promising that I would call him if there were any changes in Nancy's condition. I also let Mark know that if Nancy seemed all right, I would plan to spend the night sleeping at my girlfriend Cora's house. Because Cora lived less than a mile away, I would still be very close.

When Dr. Matthew returned later in the afternoon, I told him I was staying the night with Nancy. He argued that I needed rest, but he understood why I felt I had to stay. I did tell him I had a friend who lived nearby who could put me up, but that I would only do that if I was fairly certain Nancy was doing all right. In Dr. Matthew's opinion Nancy was doing fairly well, now that he knew her blood gases were good. He said he would see us in the morning.

I took a little break to go find something to eat in the hospital cafeteria. I didn't eat much, but at least it was something. I drank more coffee than anything. After I had eaten, I gave Cora a call. She already had plans to go out, but said she would be glad to pick me up so I could sleep over. I suggested instead that she pick me up at 9:00 a.m., so I could shower and take a break. That was fine with her. She promised to be waiting out front for me at nine.

I spent the rest of the night watching Nancy. She had only opened her eyes four or five times during the day, but each time I would tell her I loved her and that I was with her. There were no cots available in the hospital, so I sat in a rocking chair and tried to take little snoozes. Every time I would begin to doze off, the alarm on Nancy's I.V. would sound. There was nothing wrong with the I.V., but still the buzzer wouldn't stop. By 5:00 a.m., I would have been glad to sleep on the floor, but the ward was packed and there wasn't enough floor space.

Sunday, February 22, 1981

I watched the sun come up. Even though I hadn't slept, somehow I felt better. There was no change in Nancy, and my feeling was she must be getting worse. She still wouldn't drink more than a tiny sip whenever I tried to feed her. Shortly after seven, I made my way downstairs to meet Mark. When he showed up with my change of clothing, I told him there was no change. I said I would call him at work later. I let him know I was going over to Cora's to sleep for a few hours. After he was on his way, I went to the ladies' room to change, splashing cold water on my face in an effort to wake up a little.

By eight-thirty, Dr. Matthew and Dr. Willis had come in. Dr. Matthew checked Nancy and saw that she wasn't any better. "I'd say she's worse," I told him. I mentioned that she was also refusing to drink anything. His only response was to tell me to go home and get some sleep, adding that I wasn't doing any good here. I told him that I was leaving at nine. There was no need for him to tell me to leave; since he was there with Nancy I knew I had to leave anyway. I wanted to blurt out that I felt I was no good to anyone anymore, but he didn't need a weeping, babbling mother on his hands.

While Dr. Matthew was busy at the nurses' station with Nancy's chart, the nurse came in and handed me Nancy's phenobarbital (liquid) medication. I tried everything I knew to get it into her, but Nancy wouldn't cooperate and the medicine ended up all over her. In total disgust, I left her bedside. I found Dr. Matthew and told him she wouldn't take the medication, and that I had no idea what he planned to do to get it down. Dr. Matthew simply looked at Dr. Willis and said, "Rosemary is going home now to get some sleep." I said, "Okay - Bye!" and left. If there was nothing else I had learned from the past, I at least knew when I was needed and when I was not. This time, I definitely was not.

Cora was waiting for me at the front entrance, so I climbed wearily into her car and we drove off. She must have seen with one glance that I was desperate for sleep, but when we got to her house, she just chatted on and on. I listened politely, but by ten I had to say goodnight. I asked her to wake me up at noon so I could shower and get back to the hospital by 1:30 p.m. Then I went to lie down.

As soon as my head hit the pillow I was gone. The next thing I knew, Cora was coming through the door, telling me it was 12 :00 noon. I got up, put my feet on the floor, feeling like a million bucks. Cora had a hard time believing me, but I told her I had crammed eight hours of sleep into two. I took a shower and was ready to get back to the hospital.

I arrived at 1: 30 p.m., and no sooner had I walked into Nancy's room than the head nurse exclaimed, "There you are! We've been trying to get hold of you." I wanted to know what was wrong. She told me that Dr. Matthew had had to do a "cut-down" on Nancy. A cut-down is a procedure that involves going beneath the skin to find a vein. She told me that she had protested when she saw the doctors were about to perform the cut-down right there in the ward. "We've never had this done up here," she explained. "It's supposed to be done in the emergency room." (You've never had a Nancy, either, I thought).

She went on to tell me they had given Nancy her own room next to the nurses ' station so she could have privacy and a little more space. I apologized for not being available when they needed me, adding, "But I'm here now." She said, "Good! Sign these permission papers for the cut down so I don't have to worry anymore!" I laughed, and signed them without question. I explained to her what a good doctor Dr. Matthew was, and how I had perfect confidence in his judgment. She agreed, but maintained that proper procedures should still be followed. "With the kids in this place today," I cracked, "I'm surprised anything is going normal in here!" She laughed, and told me that when she got home tonight she was going to sit down with a double martini and forget the day ever happened! I told her to please have one for me. Humor was often the one thing that kept us from climbing the walls.

I went in to see Nancy in her new "private" room. When I reached her side, it was plain that Nancy wasn't doing well at all. She did respond to me, but only for a few seconds. But I was determined to keep my faith. I knew she would pull through, no matter what. I examined the cut-down they had done on her, and it looked pretty gruesome. Dr. Matthew had picked her inner left ankle to do it, and it looked really sore. By around two o'clock, Dr. Matthew arrived again. He commented that I looked much better. Then he explained the reason for the cut-down. He had been able to get the medication into Nancy, but when her vein blew, he had to remove the I.V. I wanted to know if the cut would leave a scar. He said yes it would, but explained that by the time Nancy was old enough to care about such things, it wouldn't show.

Dr. Matthew then asked me how I felt Nancy was doing. I told him it was evident to me that Nancy was in a bad way. I began to cry. He told me he would like to transfer Nancy to the UMASS ICU because Holden was not properly equipped for her. "Damn!" I said. "I don't want her there!" He said he understood my feelings, but said that if anything serious should happen to Nancy he was afraid Holden couldn't help her. Deep within I knew he was right. I explained to him that I wouldn't mind so much if Nancy were only going to the Intensive Care Unit. It was the idea of her ending up on the floor after she came out of ICU that bothered me. I admitted that I probably didn't have much of a choice, since it was Nancy who needed the care. Dr. Matthew gave me some time to think about it, saying he'd be back in a few minutes.

I gazed at Nancy and started to cry all over again. A nurse came into the room and tried to comfort me. They were all so good to us there; it was as though we were becoming family to them now. Dejectedly, I explained to her that my problem wasn't so much that Nancy had to go to the UMASS ICU floor; I knew it was an excellent unit. But I definitely didn't want Nancy on their hospital floor after she was released from ICU. The nurse replied, "So have her transferred back here after she gets out of ICU." I stopped crying and said, "What?" She repeated, plainly, that if I wanted her to come back to Holden after she was ready to leave ICU, she could finish her hospital care here. I was still thanking her when Dr. Matthew returned to see me smiling. I told him, "I will agree to the transfer if Nancy can come back here when she's ready to come out of ICU." He replied, "Sure, I'll start the paperwork and call UMASS."

Then things started rolling. Several nurses came in to prepare Nancy for the trip to UMass. The next shift was coming in just then, so there were quite a few nurses around. They could all see how happy I was, and I quickly explained why. As I stood in the doorway to Nancy's room, I suddenly turned around to see my sister-in-law Ann behind me. I quickly guided her out to the hallway to talk. All I could think of was that Nancy's cut-down was showing, and they were cleaning her up to go. I couldn't let Ann see it; she might be alarmed and not understand. I explained to Ann that Nancy wasn't at all well, and that we were in the process of transferring her to UMASS, which was the best place for her right now. I was very brief and firm, since I knew I had no time to comfort anyone right now but Nancy and myself. I told her that Mark and I would be home just as soon as Nancy was settled in at UMASS.

Dr. Matthew then came to say that he was on his way down to get Nancy's X-rays to send along with her to UMASS. Would I like to see them? I said yes, I would. As we were talking on our way down the hall, we met up with a nurse carrying Nancy's X-rays. "We're too late," Dr. Matthew said. That was okay; it was the thought that counted.

As we turned to walk back, Dr. Matthew asked me where Mark was. I answered that he was at work, but that I was about to call and let him know of the transfer because he had to pick me up. Dr. Matthew advised that I really needed somebody to talk to, someone who could help me through all this. I agreed, but I couldn't think of anybody. He told me how concerned he was that I hadn't been talking to anyone through this whole thing, and repeated that I really needed that support. Dr. Matthew knew from earlier conversations that I didn't even have the time to clean my house, and that I was virtually alone in this crisis. "Isn't there anybody who would give you support, who can help you?" he asked.

I began to cry, leaning up against the wall in the hallway. "You're the only friend I have!" I wailed. "No one understands. I don't want to go explaining my feelings to someone who can't understand what I've been through. I can't cry in front of people without explaining myself." I then added, "There is really only one person who would help me now."

"We'll get 'em!" he said. "Who is it?" "It's my sister Tina," I replied. He prompted me to call her up and have her come stay with me. I told him I couldn't bring myself to do that; she had two kids of her own and lived down in New Jersey. "So?" he demanded. I told him I couldn't expect her to pack up and leave just because of me.

"So?" he demanded again.
"I can't."
"Why?"
"I don't know."
"Don't you think she'll come?"
"Yeah, that's just the problem, she would."
"Then call her," he commanded.
"All right, I will." I felt a little better.

I was hard for me to ask for help. The way I saw it, everyone had their own problems and didn't need me to bother them. Those nearest to us seemed willing and available to help, but I was overwhelmed with the shame of imposing on them, or appearing to be crying, "poor me." It wasn't self-pity; I just wanted to handle this alone. Maybe my actions to cover over how hard it was to deal with this was coming to a head. And now it was obviously too much for me. I felt inhibited crying in front of anyone. I was sure no one would take me seriously, but just push it off, saying, "Nancy will be fine - don't worry!"

Then I'd want to yell, "Sure! She could have died on me, but how would you know-you haven't been there!"
I did need Tina. She wouldn't ask me questions or try to diagnose Nancy. I needed her just because of who she was. She was the kind of friend, who would simply come in and take charge, without my having to ask her to do anything. She would notice whatever was needed and take care of it.

The ambulance drivers passed us in the hall with the stretcher, and Dr. Matthew said that we'd better get going. He wanted to know if I had any of the five sleeping pills left that he had prescribed for me awhile back. I told him I still had two left. He instructed me to take both of them tonight just before I went to bed so I could get a good night's rest. Dr. Matthew had a call waiting for him and had to leave. As we parted, he promised to call UMASS to advise them that we were coming so they could be ready for us. "Sure," I laughed. I'd have to see it to believe it!" We both knew things didn't always run all that smoothly at "the zoo."

Nancy was all set to leave, along with a nurse from the hospital who was coming with us. We had no time to waste. I quickly asked Dr. Matthew if he wanted me to call him later. Yes, he said, he'd be waiting for my call. As we left, there were at least six nurses watching us go. I called to them, promising that we'd be back, and asking them to please save a bed for Nancy. They assured me they would.

On the way out, the Director of Nurses briefed me on everything I would need to know. She ended by asking if I had called Mark yet. No, I told her. Would she kindly call him for me right away? He would be getting out of work shortly, I explained, and unless he got the call now, he would come here and find us gone. She said she would do it right away, and told me to take care. "We'll be back," I said one last time. "Hold a bed for Nancy."

I rode in the front of the ambulance with the driver. The nurse and the EMT were in the back with Nancy, and there was no

129

space back there for three adults. I spent the time pulling my thoughts together in preparation for UMASS. I wrote a few notes to myself, carefully thinking things through as we went. I was determined to have her brought straight up to ICU, with no long stay in the Trauma Room as she had done before. I had to prepare myself for possible confrontation. I wanted to arrive as "cool, calm and collected" as possible. I prayed silently.

The ambulance driver was not wasting any time, especially after the nurse asked, "How much longer?" I knew I didn't need to panic. I knew deep down, just as I had known on Friday, that with the proper treatment Nancy was going to be all right.

When we arrived at the UMASS Trauma Center, Mark was waiting for us outside. I told him that Nancy definitely was not well. "Nobody had better fool around here," I warned him. "She'll be all right now," Mark said. Then Mark struck up a conversation with one of his acquaintances on the ambulance crew as we proceeded into the Trauma Unit.

2-21-81 U. Mass. 5th admission
"Disch. diagnosis -
1. Bilateral Pneumonia, probably viral.
2. Panhypopit. w/ controlled hypothyroidism & hypocorticism.
3. Seizure disorder, probably 2nd to hypogly.
4. Mild asthma.
5. Transient hypoglycemia.
6. Iron deficiency anemia.

It was 4:25 p.m. when we passed through the doors of the Trauma Room. The nurses on duty were plainly pregnant. They asked the ambulance crew to "put her over here on this table." "Don't move her," I commanded. They all looked at me. I repeated, "Don't move her." They were all shocked, even Mark. No one touched Nancy. The nurse who had come with her from Holden asked for oxygen for Nancy, explaining that she now had respiratory distress. The nurses all got busy

130

taking care of her. I knew I was not hysterical; I was deliberately demanding. I announced to them all that Nancy was going upstairs to the ICU and not staying down here.

Just then, the doors on the other side of the Trauma Room opened, and in walked a doctor I had never seen before. He was about average height, somewhat small in frame, and his name tag read "Family Practice Doctor." ("Okay," I thought. "Let's see what he knows.") He came over to Mark and asked, "What is wrong with her?" I gave him a blank stare and told him that they had been called ahead on Nancy. He said he knew that, but asked again what was wrong with her.

Now my blood pressure was rising. I had been through this routine four times before, and no one else except Mark knew Nancy at this point. The ambulance men were eager to leave, but couldn't go because I had not given them permission to move Nancy off the stretcher. For the first time, I had everyone 's complete attention. Now I was in control, and I wasn't going to waste it.

Speaking directly to the doctor, I demanded to know what was going on. "You were called ahead on Nancy for admission to Pediatric ICU. Here she's been transported by ambulance, with a nurse from Holden Hospital, and you want to know what's wrong with her?" By now I was screaming full force. My anger felt hysterical, but my words were direct and firm. "She has panhypopituitarism, hypothyroidism, and hypoglycemia. She also has double pneumonia. The kid is barely breathing. You'd better get moving fast and get someone from upstairs down here quick, because I'm not fooling around anymore. I want her taken care of before there are any more complications. The kid is sick enough!"

As I spoke, the doctor kept backing up. Mark took me aside, telling me to try to calm down. I told Mark that I was sorry that I had let my anger come out (because of their lack of communication skills among professionals). But I couldn't stand back and watch them play any more games with Nancy.

131

No one moved in the room. The doctor disappeared. I supposed everyone was waiting for my next move. I could tell the nurse from Holden was secretly pleased with my actions. She knew how badly Nancy needed help. Mark kept repeating, "Calm down, please calm down." 'Tm not calming down," I told him. "They're not fooling around with Nancy anymore, and if I have to get raving mad to get them to move I will. I will not wait in this room five hours or move until the shift changes."

By now minutes had passed, and a doctor that I knew ran in. She was pregnant, too. Great. Now we had three very pregnant women in here. Well, I was not going to calm down just for the sake of their condition. I directed my gaze at her and said, "Sandy, I am not fooling around this time. This girl is going upstairs as fast as you can wheel her up there. You know she's better off upstairs." Sandy replied, "Let's get some blood from her and an X-ray, then I'll take her up." She started organizing everyone to help her get Nancy off the stretcher. I glared at her and said, "Don' t move her!" All hands went off Nancy, and again, no one moved. "Nancy is going upstairs," I said firmly. "You can do all the work she needs up there; don't fool around with me." Here I had three pregnant women around me - if one started premature labor I would definitely be a cause!

Sandy suggested, "Just give me a few minutes to do these tests and then we'll bring her upstairs. It's easier to do them down here." I told her Holden had sent her X-rays, but she said they needed their own, too. I finally agreed to it, but I insisted that there would be no more than that without my permission. "A few minutes is all I'm giving you," I added, "and if I get any more trouble I want you to know that I know someone on the Board of Directors of this hospital. If you make me use him, I will. I am not fooling around this time." When I mentioned the Board of Directors, she looked directly at me, so I repeated, "Yes, I do know someone, and I will use him." I did not threaten suit because I didn't believe in it unless absolutely necessary. Making threats just wasn't part of my nature. I am not one to boast or use authority, but the time was right.

The EMTs went to move Nancy from the stretcher, then hesitated and glanced in my direction. "Yes," I responded, "you can move her now." The doctor started to get blood from Nancy. I told her Nancy had no available veins, and wished her good luck. I apologized to the nurse and the ambulance crew for detaining them, but they said it was all right. At one point, Mark had tried to convince me to let them move Nancy so the ambulance crew could leave. "You can't stop these people!" he protested. "They have to get back to the hospital." I replied that I was aware of that, but they would just have to wait.

The doctor took blood from Nancy's groin - a main artery. I was disgusted. I was so sick of needles being poked into her. Then they quickly wheeled Nancy into X-ray. When they returned soon afterward, we were immediately rushed to the Pediatric ICU. It was now 4:45 p.m., and the nurse on duty told me that we had set a record for the shortest time spent in the Trauma Unit. "Good!" I crowed. "By how much?" "Thirty minutes," she answered. I apologized to both nurses for creating a scene, but added that I had my reasons. They both understood.

While Nancy was in X-ray, I had taken the opportunity to reassure the nurses that I was not questioning their professional competence by insisting that the work be done upstairs. It was simply that it could just as easily be done up there, and I wanted Nancy under close care as soon as possible. They agreed with me, explaining that this was the way doctors do things, and they only took orders. We laughed, and one of them quipped, "Except this time, of course!" I wished them both luck with their babies and left.
In Pediatric ICU, Nancy was placed in a crib and made comfortable. Then they placed a croupette tent over her head. The croupette tent was made of plastic material and shaped

like a bowl. In contrast with the kind of tent that covers the whole body, this one provided her with direct moisture and air on her face.

> Doctors' Notes: "On admission, she had mild to moderate respiratory
> distress, with scattered wheezes bilaterally and coarse bilateral bronchial
> sounds, with only fair air exchange bilaterally. Her respiratory rate was
> between 50 - 70 per minute, and there were some subcostal and intercostal retractions."

Mark and I only needed a brief time to discuss all the information with the doctor because she already knew Nancy. I mostly had to fill her in on Nancy's recent history prior to her admission to Holden.

I added that I was sorry for my brash persistence, and she said it was all right. They all knew me from prior admissions, and although I felt somewhat badly that I had used such a forceful approach to get what I expected, I did not feel guilty in the least. However, I did deeply regret overwhelming the doctor who had greeted us in the Trauma Room. He had never seen me before that, nor did we ever see each other again.

When I went to check on Nancy just before leaving, she looked better. Her color had definitely improved, and I sensed she was going to be fine. I gave her a kiss, and told her I loved her. She was sleeping, but I knew she heard me. I told the doctor I would call later on to check on Nancy. She knew my number, and they were to call me if needed.

We arrived at Mark's mother's place at around seven-thirty and announced that Nancy was doing fine. They weren't always sure what to believe, since Nancy's episodes were so often sudden and traumatic. But truly, I knew Nancy was fine now - at least a little better than she was before. I couldn't bring myself to tell anyone how serious it had been; it wouldn't be worth it. At any rate, I told Mark about Dr. Matthew's insistence that I get someone to help me, and that I would be calling Tina. He agreed with my plan, saying we would call my sister as soon as we got home.

I knew Dr. Matthew was waiting for my call, so I contacted him from my in-laws' place. The first thing he asked was how I was doing. I reported that I was fine now, and that Nancy was settled down and looking better than she did when I first left her. He wanted to know how things had gone when we arrived at UMASS, and I described to him what I had done. All he said was, "Good!" I asked him if he thought what I had done was wrong, and he answered no, that it was the only way I could have gotten anything done. By this time I was laughing, and describing to him how thoroughly I had yelled at them. "I really did it this time," I said. Dr. Matthew had never instructed me to scream in order to get things done, but I had done what was necessary. I shared with him my discovery: the more one yelled, the faster they worked! You didn't let them fool around with your baby; you just couldn't. And they had fooled around with Nancy enough.

Dr. Matthew told me he would see Nancy in the morning. "I'll be there," I said. The first thing I did when we got home was to settle Jamie down in bed. Then I picked up the receiver and dialed Tina. When I heard her voice on the other end, I barely managed to say "Hi" before I broke down crying. I explained to her what my doctor had said about needing someone to help me. I told her that since she was my choice, he had made me promise to call her. I briefed her on the fact that Nancy was not doing well and that I hadn't been home much. The house was a mess, I confessed. Tina promised to be here by tomorrow afternoon. She merely said that she would see me when she got there. I began to stammer about being sorry, but she cut me off with, I'll see you tomorrow. Bye!"

After I finally stopped crying, Mark told me to go right to bed because I really needed the rest. I agreed, but first I wanted to call and check on Nancy one more time. The nurse at UMASS reported that Nancy was doing fine. Her respirations were the same, and she was expected to remain stable throughout the night. She said that if anything changed she would call me back. I thanked her and let her know I would be there in the morning.

By now it was ten o'clock. I swallowed the medicine Dr. Matthew had prescribed and went to bed. As always, I closed my eyes to say my prayers. I pictured Nancy lying in the crib at UMASS, with monitors on one side of her and two bottles of I.V. - one saline and one medication rigged up on the other side. Slowly I began the Lord's Prayer with "Our Father..." Suddenly, my vision of Nancy began to focus on the white wall just behind her crib. I could make out the image of someone standing there. I first saw His feet. He wore brown leather sandals. And as my eyes were lifting up, He was clothed in a pure white robe tied around the waist "With a white cord of rope. The rope was tied in front, with the two ends dangling to just below His knees. He was six feet tall. His arms were stretched out toward Nancy with palms open; there were no wounds.

As my eyes were raised, perfect peace washed over me - I had no fear of whom I was seeing. He was clean-shaven, His skin color was white, and He had medium-brown wavy shoulder-length hair parted down the middle. As I came upon His eyes, I knew who HE was. It was Jesus.

His eyes were indescribably blue - I had never seen this color blue before. They shone "With brilliance, yet they were so soft. Peace and love filled those eyes. I said to Him, "Oh! You're there." Indescribable peace flowed through me, and in a moment I was sound asleep.

Monday, February 23, 1981
I got up early so Mark could drop me off at the hospital before he reported in for work. I could hardly pay any attention to the condition of the house. It was a mess, and in my state of

physical and mental exhaustion, there was nothing I could do about it. Tina would understand. At around eight o'clock I arrived at UMASS. Nancy looked gorgeous - she really looked well. She was a bit swollen from the cortisone increase, but because I knew her so well, I could recognize her true condition well ahead of the medical staff.

Dr. Matthew came in and exclaimed, "My, you're here awful early!" I explained how I had wanted to be there for the rounds, and had not expected to see him there so early, either. Dr. Matthew took a quick look at Nancy, put his hand on her leg, and quipped, "Nancy, you're making a fool out of me." I smiled. "She does look good, doesn't she?" He told me that her latest test results looked better. I wanted to tell him all about my vision last night, but held back for fear that no one would believe me. With all the stress I had been under for the past 48 hours, I was likely to be taken for a candidate for the psych ward. For now it would have to remain between me and Jesus. I didn't know why the vision had come to me, much less how to explain it.

As Dr. Matthew got ready to leave, I asked him to let Holden know we would be on our way back there. He smiled and said okay.

Very little had to be said later when the doctors came through on their rounds. I knew them and they knew me, and we were all familiar with what had been going on with Nancy. No doctor there ever had to stand me up emotionally. I always listened to what they said. This didn't always mean I agreed, but at least I listened. Dr. Sizer told me that they would just keep a watch on Nancy now for the next few days to see how she progressed. I made sure they understood that I wanted no X-rays taken on Nancy without my prior knowledge. Dr. Sizer advised me that they would need one more before she was released from ICU, unless she failed to improve. I agreed to that, but repeated that I was to be informed. I also expressed my wish that Nancy not be transferred to the floor at all. Whenever she was released from ICU, she was to be transferred straight to Holden Hospital. I became a broken record to everyone responsible for Nancy, stating over and over again that she was to be transferred only to Holden, and not to the floor. My concern was that during the night they might decide they needed Nancy's bed, and if they thought she was well enough to leave the ICU, they might put Nancy on the floor after all. I became a constant reminder to them.

The rest of the morning went along without event right up until noon, when Nancy's I.V. infiltrated and a new one had to be started. Dr. Stem, from the clinic, had started the present one four days ago, so it had held out as long as anyone could expect.

The I.V. team was called in. When the woman arrived, she took one look at me and realized who Nancy was. The nurse was called in to help, and we all stood in suspenseful silence for the first poke. Nothing. The woman said she would try again. In the meantime, she asked me, "Who did the cut-down?" I replied that it had been done by Nancy's doctor in Holden. She wondered whether it had been necessary; but I explained that it had been a last resort to get vital medication into her, and that it had worked just long enough to succeed. She proceeded to start the I.V. once again, saying, "Let's pray this one works." I did pray - in silence. She got it. The relief on all our faces was a visible, joyful amen.

Nancy did well the rest of the day. She woke up a few times, and I knew she was continuing to get better.

After Mark had finished work, he came to see Nancy. He was glad to see how well Nancy looked. He talked for a little while with the nurse and the doctor, then we left. There wasn't much to do, since we were unable to hold Nancy or play with her. At the moment, everything had to be focused on giving her as much rest and moisture as possible. I had already spent a long day with her, and had plenty of endurance left to stay with her longer, but Mark was clearly anxious to get going. He never minded staying -with her if she was up and ready to play, but this wasn't the time for that.

When we got home at about 5:30, Tina was there. Jamie was thrilled to have her cousins to play with. Supper was all ready when we walked in, and the house looked great. It was "just what the doctor ordered!" I had to ask Tina where she had gotten the food. She told me that Mark's mother had brought a couple of bags with her when she dropped Jamie off. I explained to Tina that Mark's mother had been doing this all winter, since I never had time to go to the store! Mark added that he had asked his mother to get us something, because there wasn't much to choose from in the house. I called my mother-in-law and thanked her ever so much.

We had been eating at home, but very little. It seemed every time I sat down to make a list, something prevented me from getting to the store. I had not been eating well at all because of all my running around. Whenever I was at the hospital I practically lived on coffee. Once I had eaten a banana of Nancy' s. I had lost about ten pounds - which didn't seem like a big change until I tried my clothes on. I was definitely too thin for my build, and very drawn from all the stress. Stress always left me eating like a bird unless someone had the presence of mind to sit me down and place a prepared meal in front of me.

We enjoyed an excellent supper and relaxed for the rest of the night. As usual, before going off to bed we made our plans for the next day. Mark's mother was going to drive Jamie to see Dr. Matthew at 3:30 p.m. to get her cough treated. My other sister, Sharon, was coming over to spend the day with Tina, and I was going to the hospital. Mark would drive me over on his way to work.

Tuesday, February 24, 1981
I arrived at the hospital to find Nancy progressing beautifully. She was starting to eat more, and her respiration was responding to the bronchial treatments that she received every two to three hours. She had been put on a BRAT diet,

consisting of bananas, rice cereal, apple juice, and toast. When I fed Nancy her lunch, she took in 1/2 jar of banana/rice cereal, six ounces of apple juice, and four ounces of glucose water. She was out from under the croupette tent for three to four hours and seemed to do just fine. Dr. Sizer asked me for permission to do an X-ray on Nancy. He felt it was necessary, so I consented. Then the nurse told me that maybe tomorrow Nancy would be well enough to be transferred to the floor. The floor- I knew it! I told her firmly that Nancy was going back to Holden Hospital from ICU, and no one had better put her on the floor!

In the meantime, I received a call from Dr. Dayton, a pediatric specialist in asthma. For the past few months, Dr. Matthew had been suspecting that Nancy could have acute asthma, and it was now time to get an opinion on it. I had placed a call to Dr. Dayton on Monday, letting the doctors at UMASS know that I was asking him for a consultation.

It didn't take much time for me to update Dr. Dayton on Nancy's history; I was becoming very professional by now. Dr. Dayton told me that he planned to come in to examine Nancy. He explained that if she were wheezing before the onset of a cold, it normally would be asthma, and during a cold it was bronchiolitis. I asked him, "What is the difference between bronchiolitis, bronchitis, and bronchiectasis? He merely said that with a child, because of the young age, it was called bronchiolitis. With mature patients, it was up to the doctor which term was used. I thanked him, thinking to myself that there was nothing more confusing than to hear three different terms used for the same diagnosis!

Dr. Dayton mentioned a drug commonly used for asthmatics, but he would have to be sure Nancy's system could handle it. He added that testing could be done, but since she had been through so much recently, he wanted to wait. He would plan to see Nancy again when she was well. I promised to call him at the first sign of wheezing.

'Later on, when I spoke with the nurse, she mentioned that Nancy should be able to go to the floor tomorrow. I told her firmly that when Nancy was ready to be transferred, she was going right back to Holden. Under no circumstances was she to be moved to the floor from ICU. Dr. Sizer overheard the conversation and came into the room. I looked him in the eye and said, "Nancy will be transferred to Holden from here, right?" He smiled and answered yes. He added that Thursday was the day they planned to transfer her. I told him I would notify Dr. Matthew, and that I would be here for her transfer.

Wednesday, February 25, 1981

Tina and the girls planned to go back home today, but not before they had peeked at Nancy. I accompanied Tina to the hospital, and stayed in the hallway with her girls while she went in to see Nancy. Then the nurse came out and invited the girls in to see their cousin. Their faces beamed with smiles as we led them in to see Nancy, who was sound asleep. I was prepared to wake her, but Tina remarked how beautiful she was just lying there, and told me to let her sleep. Watching them look at Nancy brought tears to my eyes. Tina noticed and gave me a hug.

After a few precious minutes, Tina and the girls had to head home for New Jersey. I walked them down to the lobby and stayed with the girls while Tina brought the car around. It was snowing quite heavily, and I felt concern for their safety on the road. Of course, I managed to feel guilty and somehow responsible for this inconvenience, but Tina said she planned to take her time. Since they were headed south, she felt they would be out of the snow soon. We said good-bye and - as usual - I cried some more.

After they left, I headed back upstairs to spend the rest of the day with Nancy. She was back on the BRAT diet, which was made up of bananas, rice, apple juice, tea, and toast. She had never had the tea, but the doctor told me since she was doing well eating, they would take out the I.V. and transfer her to Holden tomorrow. I was thrilled. I spent the rest of the day playing with her, holding her, and feeding her.

Thursday, February 26, 1981

      1. Bilateral pneumonia, probably viral
      2. Panhypopituitarism, with controlled hypothyroidism
      and hypocorticism
      3. Seizure disorder, probably secondary to
      hypoglycemia
      4. Mild asthma
      5. Transient hypoglycemia
      6. Iron deficiency anemia

      TREATMENT: Treatment should consist of Amoxicillin,
      seven days, anhydrous Theophyllin should be
      continued in elixir form at 35 mg. pro. q. 6 hours for her
      asthma; Bronkosol should be given .2CC's. in 2.8 CC's.
      normal saline by hand nebulizer q. 3 - 4 hours p.r.n. for
      wheezing. Solucortef should be continued at the dose
      of 2.5 mg. in the morning, and 1.25 mg. p.o. b.i.D. and
      tapered to a dose of 2.5 mg. in the morning and 1.25
      mg. in the evening when wheezing is improved, or
      resolved. Fer-in-sol should be given, .4 CC's. of Fer-in-
      Sol, T.I.D. Synthroid 37.5 mg. in the a.m. and 30 mg. in
      the evening. She also should receive some chest PT q.
      4 hours."

Mark and I arrived at the hospital at about 10 a.m. for Nancy's transfer. We could have driven her to Holden in our car, but since she was still under treatment she had to go by ambulance. I reviewed Nancy's prescriptions with the doctor and signed all forms needed for the transfer. We were just thanking all the staff people for their care of Nancy when the ambulance arrived.

Right before we left, one of the nurses from the Pediatric floor asked me why Nancy wasn't being allowed to go on the floor. I told her it was my decision; I did not want Nancy on the floor and felt more at ease with her in Holden Hospital. I assured her my reasons were not based on lack of nursing care, but on the fact that their Pediatric floor was filled with really hard cases, and that Nancy, who was doing fairly well, would be better off in a small hospital. She understood and was not at all offended by my feelings. They knew that "well" cases, as compared to "hard" cases had to wait according to the severity of the patient's condition. She was happy for us.

I rode in the ambulance from UMASS to Holden. Mark took our car and met us there. When we arrived at Holden, Nancy was brought straight up to Pediatrics. Many of the nurses saw us coming in. They wore big smiles as we arrived, and the first thing I said was, "We're back!" One nurse looked me in the eye and told me that she honestly thought she would never see Nancy again. She was afraid that Nancy would never return when she left the last time. I was puzzled by this, and told her that I had been confident we would be back; I just hadn't known how long it would be. Anyway, the nurse couldn't have been happier to see her. Nancy was the talk of the hospital!

Shortly after Nancy was settled in, Dr. Matthew arrived. He was very happy to see us, and went right to work checking Nancy over and writing up his orders. Before he left, he let me know he was going to be off duty for the weekend. Dr. Friend would be on in his place, and he would see us again on Monday.

The rest of the weekend went pretty smoothly. My mother-in-law went to visit Nancy a few times, along with a few friends and relatives. In contrast, at UMASS hardly anyone had ever visited us. Despite all of Nancy's hospital admissions, I could only remember my mother and both sisters coming once each. I gave it little thought at the time. In looking back, however, I realized that I had been alone through a lot of it. Our family had stayed in close contact (to the great benefit of the phone company), but there really wasn't much anyone could do. Nancy was only an infant, and most of the time she was in ICU. At the time, my weariness and my preoccupation with each of Nancy's changing developments probably kept me from encouraging many visitors.

MARCH 1981

Sunday, March 1, 1981

Mark left for work in the morning as usual, saying that he would stop by the hospital on his way home. I planned to arrange a ride with someone so I could be at the hospital with Nancy for the afternoon. I looked forward to a morning I could spend at home treasuring Jamie's company, and to the lunch I would share with my in-laws over at their place. It turned out to be the most relaxing and restful morning I had enjoyed in months.

After the noon meal at my in-laws ' place, it was decided that I should drive my mother-in-law's car to the hospital, since no one else needed it that afternoon. At about one o'clock I kissed Jamie good-bye and headed out the door. When I arrived at the hospital, I found Nancy sitting up, playing with some toys. She looked tired and ready to nap. The nurse came over to tell me that Nancy had eaten a good lunch, and that the "chest P.T." she had done sounded good.

As the nurse began to change Nancy's diapers and to clean her up for a nap, my eyes were drawn to the cut-down on her ankle. I knew that the bandage had been changed daily at UMASS, where they always marked the bandaging tape with the current date. The stitches were still in Nancy's cut-down when Nancy had been admitted to Holden on Thursday, and it continued to need attention. I had made a mental note that her bandage was changed upon admission. But since the nurse at Holden had not dated the bandage, I had gone ahead and dated it myself that day. Now, as I examined Nancy's ankle I saw that the date I had put on the bandage was still there. That meant no one had changed it, and that most likely no one knew that I had marked it.

I asked the nurse if anyone had checked Nancy's cut-down. She looked at it with surprise; saying that she hadn't even known it was there. She assured me that she would take care of it and went for the fresh bandage and ointment to clean it. I thought to myself, "Okay, maybe they didn't know it was there, or maybe it wasn't written down, but it's up to the head nurse to know about these things. All Nancy needs now is an infection!" When the R.N. came over- a woman several years my junior - I asked her, "Has anyone checked this since Nancy came in?" "Oh, yeah," she answered, "we've been taking care of it." I kept my mouth shut after that. If the nurse wanted to lie about it, that was her decision. But I saw no reason for such deceit. I was tempted to expose her cover-up, but chose to restrain myself.

The nurse who cleaned it up was someone I trusted. We had always gotten along well. In fact, my mother had been one of her instructors during her LPN training. When Nancy had been brought in the last time, this was the nurse who couldn't believe it when Mark said, "She looks fine to me! " Now, as she was cleaning the cut-down, we shared the silent understanding that it had not been changed or checked until now.

While Nancy was napping, I went downstairs to have a coffee. The pediatric floor was still swelling with kids and I needed to get out of there for awhile. Before I could get away, the RN told me that Dr. Fine wanted to talk with me before I went home. I let the RN know that I was just going for coffee and would be back soon. She wanted to know if I would be taking Nancy home today. I replied that I would rather have her stay one more night. That way, Dr. Matthew could check her over in the morning and I could take her home after that. She said, "Okay," and quickly left.

It seemed to me that this R.N was acting a bit rude that day. It puzzled me, but I figured it must be her problem. She was pregnant and nearing the time when she would take leave from work to have her baby. She was probably just having a rough day.

When I returned from the cafeteria, Nancy was beginning to wake up. It was nice to play and spend some enjoyable time with her, but I was tired. It was a pattern: whenever I came to the hospital after a night's sleep, I would no sooner finish listening to all the reports on Nancy's progress and talking everything over with the staff than complete exhaustion would overtake me. It seemed that all I had done for months was listen and learn.

Soon Nancy and I discovered we had a surprise visitor - my dad. Boy, was it good to see him! I knew trials like this took a lot out of him; he hated hospitals. But we had a really nice time and I loved seeing him.

Soon after my dad left, Mark came. He was all smiles for Nancy. I had just begun to feed supper to her. It was a joy and a relief to see her eating so well. While her supper was in progress, we had another surprise visit - Mark's aunt and uncle. They happened to be in Worcester and had stopped in at UMASS, where they were directed here to Holden. It was a lovely surprise. They had really gone out of their way to see us, and I was thrilled.

As I finished up Nancy's feeding, Dr. Fine came in to ask me how she was doing. I told him she was doing fine, mentioning that she was eating everything but the chicken, which I suspected she didn't care for. I told him I thought she was looking a lot better, and he fully agreed. Then he said, "Well, you can take her home." I looked at him in shock and said, "Huh?" Mark piped up, "Oh, good, Nancy, you can come home now!" Everyone seemed to be smiling and happy about it except me. I told Dr. Fine that I was hoping Nancy could stay. I expressed to him how much better I would feel if Dr. Matthew could check her out in the morning before I took her. Dr. Fine replied, "No, we'll send her home tonight. I'll make an appointment for her tomorrow to see Dr. Matthew at the clinic." I said okay. He asked me to come along with him so we could review her medications before we left. Mark's aunt and uncle offered to drive his mother's car back to her so we could ride home together with Nancy.

As I walked down the hall to talk with Dr. Fine, I felt tears flowing down my face. All my fears about taking Nancy home began rising like a tidal wave inside me. I watched Dr. Fine as he began writing down Nancy's list of medications. In the middle of his scribbling, he glanced up and saw me crying. I apologized for the tears, explaining that I was afraid to take her home. He said he knew I had been through a lot with Nancy and told me he thought I had held up really well. Maybe it didn't look so at the moment, but he reassured me that I had really done well, that I would be all right. "Nancy's fine now," he added.

As he handed me the list of all her medications, I began to cry even harder.
> "Amoxicillin 125 mg. q. 6 hours
> Anhydrous Theophyllin Elixir, 35 mg. q. 6 hours
> Hydrocortisone 2.5 mg. q. a.m. and p.m.
> Synthroid 37.5 mg. p.o. q. daily
> Phenobarbital 15 mg. q. a.m. and 30 mg. q. p.m.
> Feosol Fer-in-Sol 0.6 cc p.o. q. daily.

"I already knew all the medications Nancy was on; it was the responsibility I didn't want. I was terrified of overdosing her. In addition, I had to give her the Elixicon - 1 tsp. at 6 a.m., one at 12 noon, another at 6 p.m., and one at midnight. And then there was the Amoxicillin to administer three times daily (at 6:00 a.m., 12 noon, and 6 p.m.), in addition to all her regular medications. I had no problem with her regular ones, but when I added in her 2:00 a.m. feedings, I could count on a maximum of a mere five hours of sleep each night.

The fears about all the medications were pouring through me now. I quit crying and started telling myself, "You'll make it...you'll make it." Dr. Fine ended by giving me a 10:30 a.m. appointment with Dr. Matthew for the next day.

I went back to the room to get Nancy ready. The nurse came

over to help get things rolling. When she started reviewing Nancy's medications with me, I halted her in midstream. I told her I already had them written down, saying that if I wasn't back tonight with Nancy, she would know I'd made it! She couldn't believe the list I showed her, and we had a good laugh together. All I could do was shake my head.

Discharge diagnosis:
1. Panhypopituitarism
2. Bilateral pneumonia, probably viral
3. Seizure disorder
4. Iron deficiency anemia

Monday, March 2, 1981
I survived the first night home with Nancy without overdosing her. She seemed to have a good night, and she ate well. I decided that perhaps my problem wasn't really the fear of messing up her medications, but simply the stress of remembering all the set hours of Nancy's schedule - what to give her at what time. I kept a written list for each day, checking off every dosage as it was given. Not only did I have to wake her at midnight for medication, but also again at 3:00 a.m. to give her a bottle. I had become a 24-hour nurse, with very little time left over for sleep.

Nancy and I arrived at the clinic at 10:30 a.m. to keep her appointment. I had dressed her in a pretty little frock and she looked simply adorable. The whole staff was happy to see her again. Dr. Matthew checked Nancy over and pronounced that she looked and sounded very well. He set her on the floor and gave her some cute toys to play with. Then we both sat down to chat. He wanted to know what was wrong. I began to cry, telling him how frightened I was of overdosing her because she was on so much medication. "I can't do it all," I moaned. "I can't do it. All I'm doing is medications and feedings. I just can't do it!" He said, "Okay." He began to go down the list of medicines and change a few things. The new list was:

Synthroid 37.5 mg. daily

148

Phenobarbital 15 mg. a.m., 30 mg. p.m.
Hydrocortisone 2.5 mg. a.m., 1.25 mg. p.m.
Elixicon 40 mg. 3 x day, a.m., noon, p.m.

He promised to take her off the Elixicon as soon as her wheezing improved. I felt better – much better. Dr. Matthew asked, "What else is wrong? I started crying all over again. "I need help. I can't cope with it."
"Nancy's doing fine," he assured me, "and she's all right."
I said, "No, it's me - I'm afraid of her. I don't know why. I need something. Not drugs, just help."

March 3, 1981

I went for my first therapy session with Dr. Matthew. Many tears flowed out of me as we talked. I didn't know what to do anymore; I was tired and feeling completely inadequate. I was desperately unsure of my ability to care for Nancy. Would all these crises just happen all over again? I had been told that she would be fine, but I couldn't seem to grasp the idea of her being well. Why did all this happen the way it did? Had I been overreacting, and if so, was that the reason Nancy kept winding up in the hospital?

Somehow I knew in my heart that Nancy would be all right now. I just needed a break so I wouldn't suffer a mental breakdown. In the last eleven months I had received quite an education in Panhypopituitarism. Had it not been such a rare disorder, and had there been support from others whose children had the same disorder, things might have gone more easily for me. But there was no one else with whom I could share the trials of Nancy's particular disorder. In just eleven months, I had to learn to serve as Nancy's doctor, nurse, and mother. Had I already been involved in the medical profession before she was born, perhaps I could have handled it a little more smoothly.

Over the next six weeks, I had a one-hour session with Dr. Matthew twice weekly – each Monday and Friday, with contact by phone on the Wednesdays of the first three weeks.

Therapy with Dr. Matthew proved to be a lifeline for me. I could not have opened up to a stranger. Mark was also supposed to go, but didn't - because he said he didn't need it.

On March 5, Dr. Wentworth called with the news that Nancy had been accepted by Washington for the study on Human Growth Hormone. This meant that Nancy would begin to grow, and the seizures could be expected to come under control. Dr. Wentworth had worked very hard on Nancy's protocol so she could be accepted into the study.

April 3, 1981
At 1 :00 p.m. at UMASS Medical, Nancy received her first growth hormone shot. It was a joyous day for me. They gave me instructions for administering Nancy's shots and arranged for a visiting nurse to come to help train me. I would learn how to dilute the medicine and give Nancy her shot three times weekly. Mondays, Wednesdays, and Fridays at around four o'clock was the preferred time.

April 22, 1981
I gave Nancy her shot for the first time. I readily developed an intense dislike for Mondays, Wednesdays, and Fridays.

May 27, 1981
Today was our last visit with Dr. Matthew. His internship was over and he was leaving the clinic. He was planning to take some time off, with no immediate plans to work in our locality. I asked him to please let us know if he did settle in the area so we could join his practice. Dr. Matthew would be deeply missed, but Nancy and I would go on. It would be a great loss to us, but one day I would tell Nancy just how important he was to her first year of life.ON MY OWN

June 22, 1981
At 4:02 p.m., a tornado hit my street. It blew up one house just across the street and took another nearby house off its foundation. Then it swung to the property next door to me and took a 375-foot chicken barn holding 17,000 birds. My house sustained some damage, but was left standing. We were all

home at the time. All I could do was thank God this time for His protection. That week I decided to begin attending church. At church I shared the vision of Jesus that I had received several months earlier on Sunday, February 22.

Journal of Clinical Endocrinology and Metabolism
©1991 by The Endocrine Society Vol. 72, No. 1
Printed in U.S.A.

"An Apparent Cluster of Congenital Hypopituitarism in Central Massachusetts: Magnetic Resonance Imaging and Hormonal Studies." Department of Pediatrics and Radiology, University of Massachusetts Medical School, Worcester, Massachusetts 01605.

This seven-page study was done on five infants: four males and one female. I was pleased that the study was completed, and that Nancy could be a part of it. Facts were uncovered which helped me to feel more secure about how I had handled Nancy's disability. It offered one reason "why" it may have happened to me. As the report states, "None of the patients was related, and the parents were not consanguineous. The apparent clustering suggests, therefore, the possibility of an as yet unidentified common environmental factor." And, much to our further satisfaction, Dr. Matthew returned in 1982 to set up his practice in our local area.

January, 1994
There were additional hospital admissions that will always remain in my memory. But there seems to be no need to mention them further. Nancy is now fifteen years old. She stands five feet, four inches tall. In 1984, Nancy was taken off Human Growth Hormone for three months and put on Protropin, a synthetic growth hormone. She has remained free of seizures since 1985, and has been off medication for seven years now.

Nancy is in the ninth grade and performing well. She enjoys school, chorus, voice lessons, shopping, and vacation time. Her personality is like a beam of light. She's a walking miracle. On August 7, 1994, I gave Nancy her last growth hormone shot.

1994 - ROSEMARY

I continued therapy off and on throughout the years, mostly because later hospital admissions for Nancy took a great deal out of me. But there were also deep inner problems leading to marital stress. Mark and I separated in 1985, and our divorce was final in November of 1988. After I experienced the vision of Jesus standing in Nancy's hospital room, spiritual realities took on new meaning for me. I didn't have to wonder anymore whether God loved me-I knew He did. I felt compelled to learn more about Him, about why He had visited me, and what meaning he had for my life. He washed away the regrets of the past, and gave me strength to face the future.

Three years after the vision, I made the decision to move beyond my simple profession of Catholicism into the experience of becoming a born-again Christian. Soon afterwards, I found that I much preferred to simply be known as a believer in Jesus Christ. I saw that "religion" is man-made, but that my Friend Jesus is not. I would now choose to follow Him, fellowshipping with others who knew Him and walking so that others could see His life within me.

In March of 1989, the Lord sent Randy into my life. We were married on October 7, 1989, with a large church celebration. I now had been gifted with a husband with whom to share my life, and the girls now had a stepfather to guide them. It was God who had made us a family.

Would my life have gone more smoothly if only I had listened earlier? I don't think so. 1982 was the year that was appointed for me to begin to understand, to start listening to the Lord. He has shown me freedom from inner bondage. He has given me wisdom, knowledge, and hope. He has lifted the chains of fear from my soul and has taught me to trust Him more and more as I grow in His way. I have begun to learn that life has more meaning when you "learn to listen."

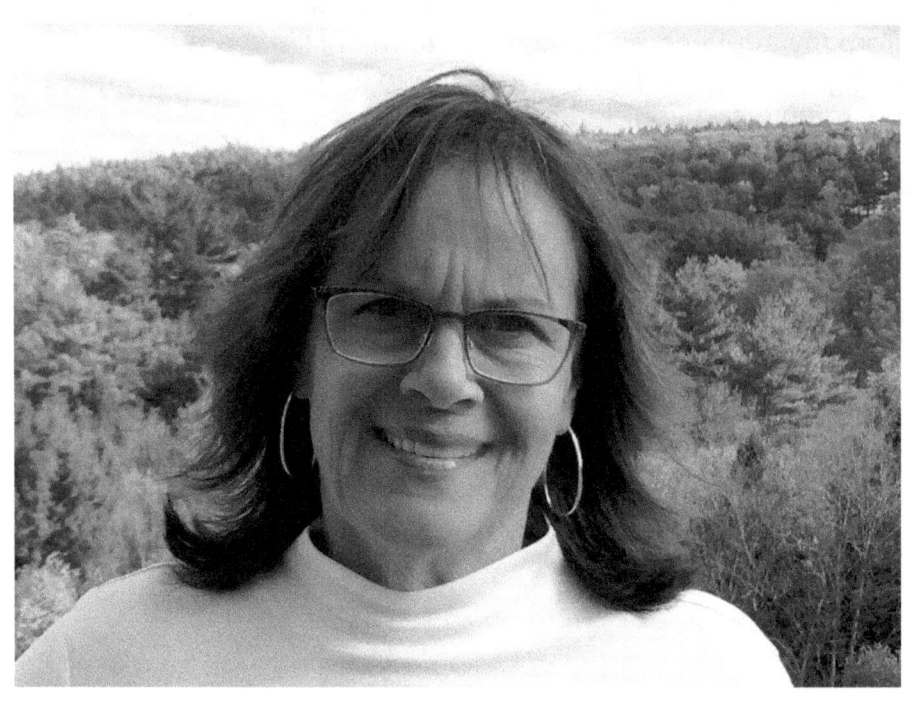

Rosemary Southwick, Author

Visit Rosemary's website iftheydonlylisten.com

For every purchase made a portion of this book will go to the CPHP Foundation http://cphpfoundation.org

*Book Cover Design by Oscar Betancur

www.ingramcontent.com/pod-product-compliance
Lightning Source LLC
Chambersburg PA
CBHW07085818O526
45168CB00005B/1866

* 9 7 8 1 5 1 7 3 4 5 2 8 0 *